The Medical Documentation
of Torture

T0297129

The Medical Documentation of Torture

Edited by

Michael Peel
MRCGP, MFOM
Senior Medical Examiner
Medical Foundation for the Care of Victims of Torture
London, UK

Vincent Iacopino
MD, PhD
Senior Medical Consultant
Physicians for Human Rights
Boston, USA

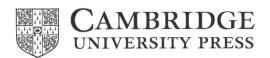

CAMBRIDGE UNIVERSITY PRESS
Cambridge, New York, Melbourne, Madrid, Cape Town, Singapore, São Paulo, Delhi

Cambridge University Press
The Edinburgh Building, Cambridge CB2 8RU, UK

Published in the United States of America by Cambridge University Press, New York

www.cambridge.org
Information on this title: www.cambridge.org/9780521117456

First published 2002
This digitally printed version 2009

A catalogue record for this publication is available from the British Library

ISBN 978-0-521-51835-2 hardback
ISBN 978-0-521-11745-6 paperback

CONTENTS

PREFACE

The forensic investigation of human rights abuses historically has focused almost exclusively on extrajudicial executions and 'disappearances'. Forensic medical involvement has been from pathologists working on the identity of victims, causes of death and the identity of perpetrators. Since the International Criminal Tribunals for Rwanda and the former Yugoslavia, many cases have focused on allegations of torture, including sexual torture. In these cases the victim is able to give a history of his or her own torture, and there are complex psychological issues. Thus the necessary skills for these new cases are different from those needed before.

Increasingly over the past 20 years, small groups of doctors and other health care professionals in a number of countries have been interviewing people who allege torture, documenting their injuries, and writing expert opinions on the validity of the claims. Initially these medical reports were compiled and used by Amnesty International as part of their reports on human rights abuses in many countries. These skills are also being used by the International Committee of the Red Cross, and the Committee for the Prevention of Torture of the Council of Europe in their investigations. Increasingly, doctors are being called on to give expert opinions on allegations of torture as part of applications for political asylum. In a few countries, such as Turkey, courageous doctors and human rights activists are providing evidence to support prosecutions of officials in criminal cases.

With more prosecutions in alleged cases of torture expected in national courts following the extradition hearings concerning Senator Augusto Pinochet in the UK in 1998–2000, and the forthcoming establishment of the International Criminal Court, there may be more opportunities for forensic medical evidence to be used. The evidence of witnesses claiming to have been tortured can be supported by an expert medical opinion that the person has physical signs and/or psychological symptoms that are, as a minimum, completely consistent with their history of torture. It must, however, always be stressed that the absence of findings does not mean that ill-treatment has not occurred. In international cases of gross human rights abuses, such medical evidence provides important evidence of torture, especially if the individuals concerned have had no contact with each other.

In 1999, more than 60 physicians, psychiatrists, psychologists, lawyers and human rights activists came together at the culmination of a three-year process to share their experiences in documenting allegations of torture and treating the victims. The result, 'The Manual on Effective Investigation and Documentation of Torture and Other Cruel, Inhuman or Degrading Treatment of Punishment (The Istanbul Protocol)', was presented to the UN High Commissioner for Human Rights, and has since been accepted by the UN for publication. It is now being translated into all the official UN languages and is expected to be available in May 2001.

The Istanbul Protocol included a set of principles that outline minimum standards for state adherence to ensure the effective documentation of torture. On 20 April 2000, the UN Commission on Human Rights unanimously annexed these principles in two resolutions (E/CN.4/RES/2000/32 and E/CN.4/RES/2000/43). These principles will be considered for UN General Assembly resolutions in the autumn of 2001. This book is a development of the Istanbul Protocol, from guidelines for the investigation of allegations of torture to an analysis of the important themes in the investigation of torture. The Istanbul Protocol is a guide of how to investigate allegations of torture, and this book explains the reasons why the medical components of such investigations should be carried out in this way. As such, it provides the foundations on which expert medical evidence of torture can be based.

Michael Peel
Vincent Iacopino

February, 2001

ACKNOWLEDGEMENT

The editors would like to thank Sherman Carroll of the Medical Foundation for the Care of Victims of Torture and Gavin Smith at Greenwich Medical Media for their help in developing the idea of this book.

CONTRIBUTORS

Kathleen Allden MD
Assistant Professor of Psychiatry
Dartmouth Medical School
Lecturer
Harvard Medical School
Medical Director
International Survivors Center
International Institute of Boston
Boston, USA

R Semih Aytaçlar MD
Chief of staff
Radiology Department
Sonomed, Istanbul, Turkey

Lis Danielsen MD
Formerly Consultant
Department of Dermato-veneriology
Bispebbjerg Hospital, Copenhagen
Consultant Dermatologist
The International Rehabilitation Council
for Torture Victims and
The Danish Rehabilitation Centre for
Torture Victims
Copenhagen, Denmark

Duncan Forrest FRCS
Senior Medical Examiner
Medical Foundation for the Care of
Victims of Torture
London, UK

Barbara A Frey JD
Adjunct Professor
University of Minnesota Law School
Previously Executive Director
Minnesota Advocates for Human Rights
Minnesota, USA

Camille Giffard LLM
Member of the Human Rights Centre
University of Essex
PhD Candidate
Faculty of Law
University of Bristol
Bristol, England

Gill Hinshelwood MBBS
Senior Physician
Foundation for the Care of
Victims of Torture
London, UK

Vincent Iacopino MD, PhD
Senior Medical Consultant
Physicians for Human Rights
Boston, USA

Robert Kirschner MD
Clinical Associate
Departments of Pathology and Pediatrics
Faculty Committee of the Human
Rights Program
University of Chicago, USA

Veli Lök MD
Professor Emeritus
Orthopedics and Traumatology
Agean University, Izmir
Delegate for the Human Rights
Foundation of Turkey, Turkey

Onder Ozkalipci MD
Forensic Physician
Human Rights Foundation of Turkey
Turkey

Michael Peel MRCGP, MFOM
Senior Medical Examiner
Medical Foundation for the Care of
Victims of Torture
London, UK

Hernan Reyes MD
Medical Co-ordinator for
Detention-related Activities
International Committee of the
Red Cross, Geneva

Visiting Research Scholar
Center for the Study of Society and
Medicine
Columbia University
New York City, USA

Sir Nigel Rodley KBE, PhD
United Nations Special Rapporteur on
Torture
Professor of Law
University of Essex
Essex, UK

Ann Somerville MA
Head
Ethics Department
British Medical Association
London, UK

James Welsh PhD
Co-ordinator of the Medical Programme
Amnesty International
London, UK

1

THE PROBLEM OF TORTURE

James Welsh

INTRODUCTION

Despite decades of intensive action by national and international human rights organisations, by the United Nations and other intergovernmental bodies, and numerous exposés by the printed and electronic media, torture persists as we start the 21st century. There remains a need for the implementation of international and national laws prohibiting the practice and for action by health workers and other human rights monitors, including the documentation and exposure of torture and other cruel, inhuman or degrading treatment. This chapter discusses the definition of torture and presents a brief introduction to the history and evolution of this abuse. It surveys the current use of torture, draws attention to some future challenges and discusses their implications for those working to end this abuse.

WHAT IS TORTURE?

Torture, as currently understood in international law, involves several elements: the infliction of *severe pain* (whether physical or psychological) by a *perpetrator* who acts *purposefully* and *on behalf of the state*. The United Nations Convention against Torture[1] defines torture this way:

> For the purposes of [the] Convention, the term 'torture' means any act by which severe pain or suffering, whether physical or mental, is intentionally inflicted on a person for such purposes as obtaining from him or a third person information or a confession, punishing him for an act he or a third person has committed or is suspected of having committed, or intimidating or coercing him or a third person, or for any reason based on discrimination of any kind, when such pain or suffering is inflicted by or at the instigation of or with the consent or acquiescence of a public official or other person acting in an official capacity. It does not include pain or suffering arising only from, inherent in or incidental to lawful sanctions (Article 1).

The World Medical Association's Declaration of Tokyo (1975), which proscribes physician involvement in torture, uses a briefer, less legalistic definition which omits the element of severity of suffering but which otherwise embodies the elements of torture cited above.

> [Torture is] the deliberate, systematic or wanton infliction of physical or mental suffering by one or more persons acting alone or on the orders of any authority, to force another person to yield information, to make a confession, or for any other reason (Preamble).

In recent years there has been growing dissatisfaction with the limited application of legal definitions, and with the protection offered by international instruments. Peters, a contemporary historian of torture, while insisting on the need to distinguish between legal and 'sentimental' definitions of torture, concedes that the definition should be expanded to take account of serious abuses permitted by law.[2] Others go further contending that grossly abusive practices carried out by individuals or groups not representing the state – that is, 'non-state actors' – should be considered in the same light as the same practices perpetrated by governments. In particular, the fact that even the most brutal domestic violence against women – arguably the predominant form of gross abuse against women – does not appear to fall within the current definition of torture, leads to a failure of international law to adequately respond to the needs of women.[3] A number of commentators argue for a reinterpretation of international law so that rape and other forms of gross violence against women might be considered as torture even where state agents are not responsible.[4] Amnesty International (AI) and other human rights monitors increasingly emphasise the duty on governments to exercise due diligence in protecting their citizens from egregious abuses even where these are not inflicted by agents of the state.[5]

For the purposes of this book, the United Nations definition serves well, provided that the experience of torture thus defined is understood to apply also to circumstances in which state agents are not necessarily the perpetrators. Thus, the infliction of severe suffering on captives by members of an opposition movement, for example, should fall conceptually within the scope of torture. This definition enlarges the perimeter in which the concept of torture is viewed while not moving too precipitately towards the 'sentimental' understanding of torture mentioned by Peters. In any event, for clinicians, the affiliation of the perpetrator of an abuse is arguably less important than the nature of the suffering experienced by the subject, its sequelae and its documentation.

While a clear understanding of the term 'torture' is important, it should not be forgotten that other forms of cruel, inhuman or degrading treatment are also contrary to international law. As with torture, cruel, inhuman or degrading treatment or punishment requires clear conceptualisation. It is obviously less severe than torture but shares other characteristics of torture: the intentional exposure of the victim to significant mental or physical pain or suffering, carried out by or with the consent or acquiescence of the state authorities. As with torture, non-state actors can inflict suffering of an equivalent type. In practice it is often less important to establish whether or not a particular act constituted torture *sensu strictu* than showing that it was contrary to laws prohibiting torture *or* other cruel inhuman or degrading treatment.[6] (Among the international standards prohibiting torture or ill-treatment are the Universal Declaration of Human Rights, the International Covenant on Civil or Political Rights, the Body of Principles for the Protection of all Persons under any Form of Detention, the Convention on the Rights of the Child and the four Geneva Conventions of 1948.)

RESURGENCE OF TORTURE IN THE 20TH CENTURY

The early history and evolution of torture – from Greek and Roman times to the 20th century – is well examined by Peters[7] and Ruthven,[8] among other authors. The key understanding of torture during the greater part of this period is that it was a part of the legal process, embodied in written laws and procedures and not regarded by states with any shame. It was viewed as a legitimate tool of investigation. This contrasts dramatically with the contemporary practice of torture where denial of any illegal acts of torture is routine; at most it may be explained away as the practice of 'rogue elements' in the police or security forces.

Despite the widely quoted view of Victor Hugo in the late 19th century that torture had disappeared – the practice was progressively outlawed in Europe between the early 18th century and the mid-19th century[9] – this was almost certainly untrue in parts of the world, where violence was endemic and where prohibitions against the use of torture were not always observed in practice. (See, for example, the account of torture in 19th century India given by Ruthven.[10])

The first half of the 20th century saw a series of struggles, usually bloody, to achieve the decolonisation of a large number of territories in Africa, Asia and the Middle East – a process which was virtually completed by the end of the century. Torture was a tool (along with bribery, persuasion, threats and other techniques) used by colonial powers to extract information which was seen as essential in maintaining control. In addition to anti-colonial wars, there were a number of serious internal conflicts between governments and opposition movements, some of which will be touched on below. The major international wars in the first 50 years of the century, notably the two world wars of 1914–18 and 1939–45, while remembered for the unprecedented scale of killing and destruction, also saw the use of torture as a tool for the gathering of intelligence. The civil wars of this period also saw torture routinely used.

However, it was during the second half of the 20th century that torture became a matter of growing public concern. From the war in Algeria in the 1950s and 1960s,[11] through the Vietnam war, the military coup in Greece in 1967 to the series of violent military coups in Latin America in the 1970s, the public was exposed to newspaper and television reports of brutality and suffering – and the protests swelled.

GOALS OF TORTURE

There are several purposes which torture can serve but the broad objectives include the maintenance of social control, the defence of ruling values and the suppression and prosecution of political opponents and criminals. In practice this means that torture is frequently used to gain information and to force confessions. In some police and security forces, torture is a short-cut to 'effective' policing through which officers can quickly gain convictions via confessions. However, torture is also used for other purposes: to disable political or social activists by intimidation or the infliction of serious trauma, to ensure compliance and collaboration from people so that they will infiltrate and/or testify against suspected 'enemies' of the government. Torture and other forms of violence can be perpetrated to assist 'ethnic cleansing' – the expulsion of one or more ethnic groups from the territory claimed by another. The social views or political stance or ideology of people who have thus been brutally tortured are immaterial to those per-petrating the torture. More generally, torture can be used to induce in a population a sense of terror. And of course, where torture has become institutionalised or where police can act with complete impunity, the threshold at which torture is seen as an appropriate tool can decrease. Moreover, torture can occur where there is no obvious purpose. There have been numerous examples recorded of individuals being arrested and tortured solely because they were, by chance, present in a location where alleged criminals or political targets of the authorities were present. No amount of torture would make them reveal information they do not have (though of course they could be induced to confess some illegal activity in which they have not participated).

Goals of torture*

Obtain information

Obtain confession

Force collaboration/co-operation/change of beliefs

Discipline/punish individuals

'Ethnic cleansing'

Spread terror in community

Self-enrichment through bribes from victims

Box 1.1

* In addition to these goal-oriented uses of torture, there are other contexts in which torture is applied: as a result of indiscipline, as a random act and as sadistic excess.

The power of torture to evoke confessions as well as to induce fear in the person under threat of torture has led some law enforcement officials to use it for their own ends. In some countries, police or prison officers have extorted money from detainees by the threat of, or actual, infliction of torture.[12] And, as Reyes has pointed out, prison guards, threatened with having their already low wages further cut if a prisoner escapes, will not hesitate to use violent forms of repression against prisoners.[13]

The targets of torture are a mix of those who have long been recognised as potential victims – foremost, political or military opponents of the ruling power – as well as others who are under-recognised as targets for torture: alleged criminals, the poor and marginalised, ethnic minorities[14] (both in their country of origin and as asylum seekers). Some victim groups do not fit into traditional understandings of political torture: sexual minorities,[15] religious groups, women and children (particularly vulnerable when used as a weapon against male family members),[16] civilians caught in civil wars or in conflicts across borders, and 'accidental' victims – those who are arrested because they have the misfortune to be in a place where security agents are carrying out arrests.

Targets of torture

Political or military opponents

Alleged criminals

Poor and marginalised

Ethnic minorities

Sexual minorities

Religious groups

Asylum seekers or immigrants

Women and children

Civilians in civil, or cross-border, wars

Incidental victims ('in wrong place at wrong time')

Box 1.2

MEDICALISATION OF TORTURE

One striking aspect of torture as practised over the past 30 years has been the participation – some time willing, some times coerced – of health professionals. In the early 1970s, reports reached Western journalists that political dissidents in the Soviet Union were being incarcerated in mental hospitals solely on the basis of their political opinions. While so held, many were subjected to ill-treatment including the forcible administration of drugs and constriction of the body in wet canvas which shrank on drying.[17] This ill-treatment, inflicted under the supervision of forensic psychiatrists, was cruel, caused great suffering and was not medically indicated. The All-Union Society of Psychiatrists and Neuropathologists withdrew from the World Psychiatric Association in 1983 when it became clear that it was likely to be expelled for tolerating the abusive use of psychiatry in the USSR. This effectively marked the beginning of the end for Soviet psychiatric abuse.[18]

Latin America

The torture which took place in several countries in Latin America from the early 1960s to the mid-1980s was systematic, brutal and medicalised. In Argentina, Brazil,

Chile and Uruguay, torture was carried out by security agencies often with the assistance of medical personnel. The reliance on medical personnel appeared to reflect both a more 'scientific' approach to the extraction of information (including the resuscitation of victims who were at risk of death under torture as well as the application of medical skills to the cover-up of the effects of torture and the issuing of false medical or death certificates).[19] The sole doctor convicted of torture in any of these countries, Dr Jorge Berges (Argentina), was sentenced in 1986 to four years' imprisonment for involvement in torture during the 'dirty war' but was released the following year under the law of due obedience.[20]

While the persistent reports of medical participation in torture and ill-treatment (and its cover-up) are alarming and deserving concerted action, it should be remembered that in many countries police and military officers have no need of doctors to assist in torture and hold no fears for the visibility of injuries on the victim or even the victim's death. They are protected by a pervasive impunity. Medical participation or acquiescence therefore has to be seen as part of the problem but not divorced from it.

DEVELOPMENT OF A CAMPAIGN AGAINST TORTURE

AI launched the first international campaign against torture in December 1972.[21] The campaign focussed on alerting the public to a phenomenon which was not sufficiently recognised and sought appeals from members of the public to governments calling for an end to torture. A report analysing the subject was published [22] and this examined legal, political and psychological factors in the use of torture and reported on the pattern of torture worldwide. The year-long campaign ended with an international conference on torture in Paris in December 1973. Workshops at the conference made a number of recommendations including several relating to the role of doctors in preventing or opposing torture.[23]

In 1984, AI started a second global campaign against torture. The campaign was based on a worldwide survey of torture and the campaign report [24] advanced arguments and tools for the protection of detainees from torture. Foremost among these tools was AI's *12-point programme for the prevention of torture.* This set out the key measures, which would make control and elimination of torture possible. These included the placing of limits on incommunicado detention, an end to secret detention, the implementation of safeguards during interrogation and custody, the independent investigation of reports of torture, an end to the use of statements extracted under torture, and a prohibition of torture in law.[25]

The campaign added weight to pressure for the adoption of the then Draft Convention against Torture, which was adopted by the United Nations General Assembly in December 1984 and came into force in 1987.

MEDICAL ETHICS AND TORTURE[26]

The roots of an ethical position against medical involvement on torture can be found as early as 500 BC in the writings of Hippocrates which underlined the primacy of the patient's well-being. However, for centuries (albeit poorly documented), some physicians and surgeons have worked on behalf of the authorities in the care and interrogation of prisoners and have, where the death penalty has been imposed, assisted in their execution.[27]

No national code of medical ethics seriously addressed the issue of torture in the period from the establishment of the first professional bodies in the 19th century until the mid-20th century. The development of modern ethics relevant to torture can be traced to the egregious abuses carried out during the Nazi period in Germany. In 1947, the newly established World Medical Association placed a high priority on stating the ethical principles which should govern medical practice and which, in particular, should make clear that all human beings had the same rights and should be treated equally. The Declaration of Geneva, adopted 1949, was essentially a re-working of the Hippocratic Oath. It enjoined doctors to 'maintain the utmost respect for human life' and 'not [to] use ... medical knowledge contrary to the laws of human-ity' though did not specifically come to grips with torture.[28]

In the subsequent two decades – and particularly in the light of alleged medical participation in torture in Latin America – it became clear that general Hippocratic principles did not explicitly address the issue of torture. In 1975, the World Medical Association adopted the Guidelines for Medical Doctors Concerning Torture and Other Cruel, Inhuman or Degrading Treatment or Punishment in Relation to Detention and Imprisonment known as the Declaration of Tokyo. This prohibited participation in torture in unambiguous terms:

> The doctor shall not countenance, condone or participate in the practice of torture or other forms of cruel, inhuman or degrading procedures, whatever the offence of which the victim of such procedures is suspected, accused or guilty, and whatever the victim's beliefs or motives, and in all situations, including armed conflict and civil strife (Article 1).

This code remains the strongest statement of the organised medical profession against participation in, or tolerance of, torture.

The United Nations likewise moved to address the persistent problem of participation by health professionals in human rights abuses and adopted in December 1982 the Principles of Medical Ethics which state that it is:

> 'a gross contravention of medical ethics, as well as an offence under applicable inter-national instruments, for health personnel, particularly physicians, to engage, actively or passively, in acts which constitute participation in, complicity in, incitement to or

attempts to commit torture or other cruel, inhuman or degrading treatment or punishment.' (Principle 2).

However, what the doctor should *do* on discovering unethical behaviour on the part of a colleague or if the doctors themselves should come under pressure to participate in abuses is not made clear, other than refraining from participating. The implication of the Declaration of Tokyo's injunction not to 'countenance [or] condone' torture or ill-treatment is that unethical behaviour by a colleague, or pressure to behave unethically, should be reported to an appropriate person or organisation. However, specific guidance is lacking (though support for doctors who do protest is given, *generally* in the Declaration of Tokyo (Article 6) and *specifically* in the World Medical Association's Declaration Concerning Support for Medical Doctors Refusing to Participate in, or to Condone, the Use of Torture or Other Forms of Cruel, Inhuman or Degrading Treatment (1997)).

Other professions also addressed the ethics of participation in torture by their own members. In 1975, the International Council of Nurses (ICN) adopted a statement on the responsibility of nurses in the care of prisoners and detainees which proscribed participation in torture.[29] The ICN went on to adopt a number of human rights declarations including revisions of the 1975 declaration as well as statements on the nurse and torture, and capital punishment.[30] The ICN declarations do give guidance on what the nurse should do when confronted with torture though the advice to nurses knowing of torture to 'take appropriate action to safeguard [the victim's] rights including reporting the matter to appropriate national and/or international bodies', present in the 1975 code,[31] was revised in 1998 to urge the nurse simply to 'take appropriate action'.[32] This drafting change is not likely to have been accidental and probably reflects a consensus within the Council that action is needed on torture but a lack of certainty about what should be done by the individual nurse; other ICN statements underline the need for national nursing associations to provide a mechanism to assist nurses aware of torture.

The World Psychiatric Association adopted (in 1977) the Declaration of Hawaii which proscribed participation by psychiatrists in what might be called 'political psychiatry' – the use of psychiatry to detain and punish opponents of the state or others who are committed to an institution for non-medical reasons. It later adopted a general statement on ethics – the Declaration of Madrid, 1996 – with specific paragraphs addressing issues such as torture.

CONTEMPORARY TORTURE

Torture practised today is either state policy – the deliberate use of torture with the tacit or open support of the government – or it can arise out of ineffective control of the law enforcement agencies, including impunity for those who carry out torture. It is also practised in conflict zones, including members of armed opposition groups. This is not new, though the understanding of the targets and context of torture is widening.

In October 2000, AI launched a renewed year-long campaign against torture. Whereas the earlier campaigns had attempted to put torture on the international political agenda and emphasised preventive mechanisms, the new campaign started from the recognition that 'there is no shortage of information on how to prevent torture'.[33] The campaign put a focus, therefore, on two issues which are central to contemporary torture: *discrimination* based on gender, social status and other factors, and the *impunity* routinely given to perpetrators.

The report issued to launch AI's campaign[34] states that torture continues to be used as an instrument of political repression as well as for other purposes. The scale of the problem is massive: AI has received reports of torture and ill-treatment inflicted by state agents in over 150 countries since 1997. In more than 70 countries, torture or ill-treatment by state officials was widespread and in over 80 countries people reportedly died as a result. However, the organisation's global survey of torture strongly suggests that the most common victims of torture and ill-treatment are convicted criminals and criminal suspects. This has serious implications for the elaboration of protective measures to prevent torture, for mobilising public opinion, for effectively ending impunity and for the wider inculcation of a culture of human rights in society. There is a serious risk that an end to political torture may take the issue off the agenda but not end the practice. As one human rights monitor stated in 1996 with respect to Brazil: 'The end of the military dictatorship was by no means an end to the practice of torture [and] torture against poor, darker-skinned people is routinely practised'.[35] The AI report makes clear that discrimination is a key element in contemporary torture. Marginalised populations, ethnic and sexual minorities, immigrants, all appear to be at an elevated risk of torture.

CHALLENGING IMPUNITY

As mentioned above, only one doctor was ever successfully prosecuted for torture during two decades of human rights violations in Latin America. The number of police or security officers prosecuted around the world for inflicting torture on detainees has been and is likely to remain very small. However, there have been some significant developments in the last years of the 20th century. These include the work of several truth commissions; the establishment and functioning of the International Criminal Tribunals of Former Yugoslavia and Rwanda in 1993 and 1994 respectively, the adoption in July 1998 of a statute for an International Criminal Court and individual attempts at prosecution of figures alleged to have been responsible for torture.

A number of truth commissions have been established in the wake of periods of undemocratic government and widespread human rights abuses.[36] One of the most recent of these was the South African Truth and Reconciliation Commission (TRC) which, like several earlier commissions, was established as part of a transitional deal which would allow the transformation of South Africa from a racist state to a democratic state. In common with virtually all commissions of its type, the TRC did not assemble evidence for use in the prosecution of torturers. On the contrary, its commitment to the 'reconciliation' component of its function meant that violators of human rights could apply for an amnesty for any crimes committed in pursuit of political goals. The trade-off for establishing the Commission was, in the view of Commissioner Wendy Orr, a simple but controversial one: 'no amnesty, no TRC'.[37] Thousands of pages of testimony were taken in TRC hearings and assessments for compensation undertaken. Perpetrators of human rights violations were given the opportunity to apply for amnesties which could only be given where applicants carried out abuses for political ends and provided that they gave a full account of their activities. This led to detached, almost surreal, exchanges of the following kind (between Ashley Forbes, a former detainee, and Jeffrey Benzien, an applicant for amnesty):

> Forbes: Do you remember ... that my clothes were removed and that the wet bag method was again used on me.
> Benzien: I would concede it could have happened.
> Forbes: Do you remember after that, putting me onto a chair and then saying to me that you are going to break my eardrum and then hitting me against my ear?
> Benzien: No, sir. Not saying I am going to break your eardrum. I gave you a smack that evening on your ear and days later you told me that you thought your eardrum was broken.
> Forbes: Do you remember saying that you are going to give me a blue eye and then hitting me against my eye?
> Benzien: No sir ... [to court:] I knew he had to be examined by a doctor.
> Forbes: Do you remember saying that you are going to break my nose and then putting both your thumb into my nostrils and pulling, until blood came out of my nose?
> Benzien: I know you had a nose bleed. I thought it was the result of the smack I gave you.
> Forbes: Do you remember choking me ... ?[38]

The TRC did not solve South Africa's problems in making the transition from apartheid to democracy and its success in balancing the conflicting goals of truth and reconciliation remain to be assessed. It did however reveal a huge amount of information about gross and systemic violations of human rights[39] as well as giving rise to important analysis both of general human rights issues and of the role of the professions during apartheid.[40] Attempts to address abuses involving members of the medical profession in South Africa, including participation or acquiescence in torture, have been thwarted by a reluctance or inability of medical institutions to address their failings. In particular there is a strong possibility that many doctors who assisted in the perpetration of human rights violations could still be practising medicine.[41]

In October 1998, the former Chilean leader Augusto Pinochet was served with provisional arrest warrants in London and held in custody pending legal proceedings at the request of Spanish judges. There followed more than a year of legal proceedings in English courts which upheld the liability of Pinochet to extradition to answer charges relating to abuses allegedly committed at his instigation and during his period of rule in Chile. Although courts consistently ruled against Pinochet's immunity to extradition, he was allowed to return to Chile on health grounds in March 2000, following a decision by the British Home Secretary, Jack Straw. The Home Secretary said he made his decision in the light of the findings of a panel of medical specialists though there was dispute about the adequacy of the panel's expertise and complaints about the lack of transparency of the procedures used.[42] On arrival in Chile, proceedings were started to prosecute Pinochet for abuses carried out during the period of his government and in January 2001 he again was examined by Chilean medical specialists. At the time of writing this has not been resolved. In March 2001 a Santiago appeals court upheld the indictment of Augusto Pinochet for human rights abuses committed shortly after the 1973 military coup, but reduced the charges from responsibility for the murder and kidnapping of opponents to being an accessory in the covering up of the crimes. Consequently, he was released from house arrest. The case is proceeding at time of writing.

Other alleged perpetrators of human rights violations were pursued by legal means. In July 1999, judicial authorities in France opened proceedings against Ely Ould Dha, an officer in the Mauritanian army, arrested while attending a course in Montpellier, after two Mauritanian political exiles filed a complaint against him before the French courts, with the support of the Fédération Internationales des Ligues des Droits de l'Homme (FIDH, International Federation for Human Rights) and the Ligue des Droits de l'Homme (LDH, Human Rights League, France). However, he fled to Mauritania before a court could determine his guilt or innocence. On 26 January 2000, a coalition of national and international human rights groups filed a criminal complaint in Dakar, Senegal, against the former president of Chad, Hissein Habré, for alleged crimes under international law (including torture) committed during the period of his rule, 1982–90. On 28 January 2000, a Senegalese judge ruled that a judicial investigation into Hissein Habré's complicity in acts of torture should proceed. However, in July 2000, a Senegalese court ruled that it had no jurisdiction to prosecute Hissein Habré for crimes committed in Chad. The coalition of non-governmental organisations (NGOs) lodged an appeal against this decision. In November 2000, the court ruled that it was not competent and although further legal procedures are before the court, Hissein Habré remains at liberty.

The Pinochet and other cases have been a major positive development in the legal pursuit of torturers. The fact remains, nevertheless, that torturers and those who protect them are likely to be at minimal risk of prosecution and conviction, at least in the short term. This remains a major challenge for human rights advocates.

LOOKING FORWARD

The circumstances which give rise to torture will not disappear in the short term. Increasingly sophisticated torture will occur along with old-fashioned brutality and violence. In some countries there may be a growing realisation on the part of those who inflict torture of the need not to leave evidence and this could mean less reliance of severe physical methods of torture (or using physical methods which leave little evidence) as well as more emphasis on psychological methods. At the same time there will be a growing capacity of NGOs and others to document torture through specialised medical evaluations but also through more effective assessment of testimony and psychological assessment. There is a risk that the result of the contest between torturers using less physically damaging torture methods and medical specialists using increasingly sophisticated forensic techniques – a torture 'arms race', in the words of one commentator[43] – will be a progressive increase in the burden of proof being placed on medical witnesses. The experience in Turkey suggests that there is a real risk that expert clinical assessment of injuries will be disregarded in favour of technically sophisticated laboratory tests;[44] there may also be a downplaying of psychological evidence.[45]

The continuing large-scale movements of populations for reasons of war, human rights abuses, and famine or other natural disasters, as well as the movement of those seeking better economic opportunities outside their own country, will place further pressure on asylum processes. The reaction in the recent past in affluent countries taking in people from such groups has ranged from tolerance to serious hostility, and misleading information has been published in the popular press with the result that anti-immigrant sentiments have been inflamed. Should this trend continue, there may be implications for the willingness of immigrants, particularly those without appropriate permits or documentation, to make themselves visible including by seeking help in public health clinics. The countries bearing the most weight of the various refugee crises are, as usual, the countries contiguous to the trouble spot. In these countries, torture documentation and issues of redress give way to the basic needs of large displaced populations and humanitarian organisations struggle to meet the needs of vulnerable populations.[46]

There is a need for the implementation of a programme of regular inspections of places of custody, a system similar to that practised by the Committee for the Prevention of Torture of the Council of Europe.[47] The International Committee of the Red Cross already plays an important role in observing, documenting and reporting to governments on prison conditions[48] but can be, and is, refused entry into some countries where its presence would be of considerable value to prisoners. The Optional Protocol of the Convention against Torture continues to attract signatories but its adoption and implementation remains far off, particularly with respect to the countries where prisoners are most at risk. Continued pressure for states to sign and ratify the optional protocol is required.

Medical professionals involved in the medico-legal documentation of torture may face either the failure of courts to admit medical evidence – in some countries only medical evidence from a qualified forensic practitioner may be admitted – or the rejection by courts and tribunals of evidence not based on gross physical evidence of ill-treatment. In Turkey, the Human Rights Foundation has reported in 1999 that even expert medical opinion concerning inflammation or scarring on the body produced by electrical torture has not been adequate for courts which seek more 'scientific' documentation. In some cases the production of sophisticated medical evidence of particular forms of torture appears to have resulted in changes to the methods of torture used – a victory of sorts but one which has not resulted in the ending of torture.[49] A more typical problem does not relate to the quality of the examination and medical findings but rather its absence. Forensic doctors in Turkey have been subjected to serious intimidation and health personnel have been attacked. Doctors involved in human rights documentation and medical care for people who have been tortured have themselves been harassed.[50] The effective medical documentation of torture requires several factors: training, competence and professionalism are certainly important factors but other pre-requisites include a framework of respect for the rule of law; guarantees of security and independence for practitioners, witnesses and complainants; openness of courts to receive and weigh medical evidence in arriving at judgements; control of police and willingness to prosecute alleged torturers. The Istanbul Protocol[51] recognises the importance of this aggregation of pre-conditions and recommends measures by which a government's commitment to uncover the truth about torture could be judged. It also provides a framework for the application of expert medical, scientific and psychological skills in the documentation of torture, as this book testifies.

CONCLUSION

Torture is an abomination which should be eradicated. The most recent evidence available suggests that torture remains a widespread global phenomenon. Victims can be political activists, or those not active in politics, male or female, able-bodied or disabled, young or old. Social marginalisation, discrimination, and conflict are the background elements giving rise to the contemporary use of torture and impunity is the key to the continuation of the practice. Discriminatory practices and attacks on the marginalised are arguably less simple to combat than the persecution of individual high profile political activists who are able to mobilise (or have mobilised on their behalf) national and international support. The coming decade will pose a challenge on this front.

International legal initiatives including the proposal for an international system of inspection (the Optional Protocol to the United Nations Convention against Torture) and the adoption of the statute for an International Criminal Court have opened up new perspectives on the future detection and prosecution of torture, though campaigning and documentation by NGOs will remain of the utmost importance. In this regard, medical documentation of torture is fundamental to the struggle for the elimination of this abuse and the Istanbul Protocol marks an important stepping stone in this quest.

REFERENCES

1   This and all other international instruments and codes of ethics cited in this chapter can be found in Amnesty International. Ethical Codes and Declarations Relevant to the Health Professions. 4th revised edn. London: Amnesty International, 2000

2   Peters E. Torture. Expanded edn. Philadelphia: University of Pennsylvania Press, 1996. By 'sentimental', Peters means the application of the term 'torture' to signify 'the infliction of suffering, however defined, upon anyone for any purpose – or for no purpose' (p 2)

3   Mainstream human rights organisations are now joining women's organisations to address this deficit. See for example: Amnesty International. Pakistan: Violence against women in the name of honour. AI Index: ASA 33/017/1999; Human Rights Watch. A Matter of Power: State Control of Women's Virginity in Turkey. New York: HRW, 1994; the creation of the Special Rapporteur on violence against women (by resolution 1994/45 of 4 March 1994) has also given an impulse to the defence the rights of women, including matters relating to the infliction of injuries in the private sphere

4   Evolving international law establishes that rape by agents of the state constitutes torture. See: Strumpen-Darrie C. Rape: a survey of current international jurisprudence. Human Rights Brief 2000; 7(3):12. See also: Copelon R. Intimate terror: understanding domestic violence as torture. In: Human Rights of Women: National and International Perspectives. Philadelphia: University of Pennsylvania Press, 1994, pp 116–152

5   See Amnesty International. Respect, protect, fulfil – women's human rights. State responsibility for abuses by 'Non-State Actors'. London: AI Index: IOR 50/01/00, 2000

6   Rodley discusses at length the definition of torture and the threshold between torture and cruel, inhuman or degrading treatment. (Rodley NS. The Treatment of Prisoners Under International Law. 2nd edn. Oxford: Clarendon Press, 1999.) For a discussion of the work of the European Committee for the Prevention of Torture see: Evans MD, Morgan R. Preventing Torture: A Study of the European Convention for the Prevention of Torture and Inhuman or Degrading Treatment or Punishment. Oxford: Clarendon Press, 1999. For a guide to the reporting of torture or ill-treatment see: Giffard C. The Torture Reporting Handbook. Colchester: Human Rights Centre, University of Essex, 2000. By contrast to the legalistic precision of international law, those who use torture employ a variety of euphemisms and slang terms to describe their practices. See: Crelinsten RD. In their own words: the world of the torturer. In: Crelinsten RD, Schmid AP (eds). The Politics of Pain. Torturers and Their Masters. Leiden,

PIOOM, 1993, pp 39–72; Feitlowitz M. A Lexicon of Terror: Argentina and the Legacies of Torture. Oxford: Oxford University Press, 1998

7   Peters E. Torture. op. cit.

8   Ruthven M. Torture: The Grand Conspiracy. London: Gollancz, 1978

9   Peters, ibid. 90–91

10 Ruthven, op. cit.

11 Vidal-Nacquet P. Torture: Cancer of Democracy: France and Algeria 1954–62. Harmondsworth: Penguin, 1963

12 Welsh J, Rayner M. The 'acceptable enemy': torture in non-political cases. Torture 1997; 7:9–14

13 Reyes H. Torture and its consequences. Torture 1995; 5:72–76

14 While ethnic minorities are vulnerable to discrimination and ill-treatment at the hands of forces of the majority population, in some countries it has been the minority which perpetrates abuses (South Africa being the outstanding example)

15 Amnesty International. Crimes of Hate, Conspiracy of Silence: Torture and Ill-treatment Based on Sexual Identity. London: Amnesty International, 2001

16 Man N. Children, Torture and Power: The Torture of Children by States and Armed Opposition Groups. London: Save the Children, 2000; Amnesty International, Hidden Scandal, Secret Shame: Torture and Ill-treatment of Children. London: Amnesty International, 2000; Amnesty International. Broken Bodies, Shattered Minds. Torture and Ill-treatment of Women. London: Amnesty International, 2001

17 Bloch S, Reddaway P. Russia's Political Hospitals, London: Gollancz, 1977; Bloch S, Reddaway P. Soviet Psychiatric Abuse: The Shadow Over World Psychiatry. London: Gollancz, 1983

18 Cases of political use of psychiatry are alleged to have arisen in other countries, most recently a small number of cases in China. See: Munro R. Judicial psychiatry in China and its political abuses. Columbia J Asian Law 2000; 14:1–128

19 Bloche MG. Uruguay's Military Physicians: Cogs in a System of Terror. Washington DC: AAAS, 1987; Stover E. The Open Secret: Torture and the Medical Profession in Chile. Washington DC: AAAS, 1987

20 In 1995, Dr Berges re-entered the spotlight when he was charged with baby trafficking as a result of his supervising births of babies from numerous female 'disappeared' – a crime not covered by the government amnesty. However, the main charges were dropped in late 1995. In 1996, Berges was shot in the street and seriously, though not fatally, wounded by gunmen claiming to be part of a previously unknown group (Feidlowitz, 1998)

21 Many national and international campaigns against political targets such as wars and colonialism had been organised in the 19th and 20th centuries. However, the 1972 campaign of Amnesty International was the first campaign specifically directed against torture which was international both in participation and in target

22 Amnesty International. Report on Torture, revised edn. London: Duckworth, 1975

23   Several of the recommendations made by the conference were promptly realised –
     one example was the recommended prohibition on medical participation in
     torture which was later embodied in the World Medical Association's
     Declaration of Tokyo, adopted in 1975. Another outcome of the conference was
     the establishment in Copenhagen the following year of the first AI medical
     group. Amnesty International. Report of the Conference for the Abolition of
     Torture. London: Amnesty International publications, 1974

24   Amnesty International. Torture in the Eighties. London: Amnesty International,
     1984

25   The 12 point program was revised in 2000 as a program for the prevention of
     torture 'by agents of the state'; see Amnesty International. Take a Step to Stamp
     Out Torture, 2000

26   See also: Somerville A, Reyes H, Peel M. Doctors and torture, Chapter 4

27   One Dutch physician who – exceptionally – opposed participating in the perse-
     cution of witches in the Netherlands in the 16th century gave his name to a
     human rights group in the late 20th century. The Johannes Wier Foundation,
     based in Amersfoort, Netherlands, is a human rights organisation comprising
     physicians and other health workers

28   This, and the other codes cited in this section, are reproduced in: Amnesty
     International. Ethical Codes and Declarations Relevant to the Health
     Professions. 4th revised edn. London: Amnesty International, 2000

29   This statement and several others were revised in subsequent years. See Amnesty
     International. Ethical Codes and Declarations ... ibid.

30   Ibid.

31   ICN. The Nurse's Role in the Care of Detainees and Prisoners, 1975 revised
     1991. See Amnesty International. Ethical Codes and Declarations Relevant to the
     Health Professions, 3rd edn. 1994

32   ICN. The Nurse's Role in the Care of Prisoners and Detainees, 1998

33   Amnesty International. Take a Step to Stamp Out Torture. London: AIP,
     2000, p 6

34   Amnesty International, ibid

35   Quoted in Hayner PB. The contribution of Truth Commissions. In: Duner B (ed.).
     An End to Torture: Strategies for its Eradication. London: Zed Books, 1998, p 216

36   Hayner P. Fifteen Truth Commissions. Human Right Quarter 1994; 16:597–675

37   Orr W. From Biko to Basson. Saxonwold: Contra Press, 2000, p 89

38   Orr W, ibid.

39   TRC. Truth and Reconciliation Commission of South Africa Report, Cape
     Town: TRC, 1998, Five volumes

40   See, e.g. Baldwin-Ragaven L, de Gruchy J, London L. An Ambulance of
     the Wrong Colour. Cape Town: UCT Press, 1999. This is based on a lengthy
     submission to the TRC health sector hearings in June 1997 made by the Health
     and Human Rights Project, a joint initiative of the Trauma Centre for Victims

of Violence and Torture, and the Department of Community Health, University of Cape Town

41   Dr Wouter Basson, on trial on charges relating to the conduct of South Africa's chemical and biological warfare programme during the apartheid years remains a registered doctor at the time of writing

42   The main point made by critics of the medical panel (who did not have access at that time to the medical report) was that the panel did not include a psychogeriatrician. The other panel members were eminent specialists. The medical report subsequently appeared translated in full in Spanish newspapers and subsequently back into English in the London. Independent, 16 February 2000

43   Jacobs U. Psycho-political challenges in the forensic documentation of torture. Torture 2000; 10:68–71

44   Turkish doctors participating in a meeting in Istanbul, March 1999, reported their experience that some local courts would not accept medical opinion concerning the traumatic origin of skin lesions but would accept cytopathological or scintigraphic findings

45   Jacobs, op. cit.

46   Medecins sans Frontieres. Populations in Danger. London: John Libbey, 1995

47   The structure and work of the CPT is described in its first annual report: 1st General Report on the CPT's activities covering the period November 1989 to December 1990. Strasbourg: CPT/Inf (91) 3 [EN], 20 February 1991

48   Staiff M. Visits to detained torture victims by the ICRC. I. Management, documentation and follow-up. Torture 2000; 10:4–7

49   In Turkey, when doctors in Izmir were consistently able to demonstrate the use of falanga the practice was ended and other methods of torture used against detainees. This kind of effective exposure of abuses pre-supposes that medical evidence is assembled by doctors in an expert and impartial way. As a report by Physicians for Human Rights showed (Torture in Turkey and its Unwilling Participants. Boston: PHR, 1996) forensic doctors in Turkey come under severe pressure not to report signs of torture. Much of the compelling medical evidence of torture in Turkey is produced by doctors working for human rights organisations – activities for which they risk harassment by the authorities

50   Amnesty International. Harming the Healers. Human Rights Violations Against Health Personnel. London: ACT 75/01/00, 2000. British Medical Association. The Medical Profession and Human Rights: Handbook for a Changing Agenda. London: Zed Books, 2001, Chapter 4, pp 56–96

51   Istanbul Protocol: Manual for the Effective Documentation of Torture. Submitted by an *ad hoc* group of medical, legal and human rights experts to the United Nations High Commissioner for Human Rights, Mary Robinson, on 9 August 2000. For background, see: Iacopino V, Özkalipçi Ö, Schlar C. The Istanbul Protocol: international standards for the effective investigation and documentation of torture and ill-treatment. Lancet 1999; 354:1117. The full protocol is available at the web-site of Physicians for Human Rights: http://www.phrusa.org

2

THE APPROACH OF INTERNATIONAL TRIBUNALS TO MEDICAL EVIDENCE IN CASES INVOLVING ALLEGATIONS OF TORTURE

Camille Giffard, Nigel Rodley

INTRODUCTION

The Istanbul Protocol sets out guidelines for medical evaluations of torture and ill-treatment.[1] It draws on the experience of a large number of medical and other professionals as to the most appropriate form and conduct of medical examinations and reports for the purpose of investigating allegations of torture. When it comes to submitting medical reports in cases before international tribunals, however, how do the tribunals themselves choose to approach the matter of medical evidence? What role, if any, does such evidence play in their decisions? Is it possible to identify distinct factors which influence the tribunals in attributing weight to particular items of medical evidence or does it all ultimately depend on the facts of the case? This chapter seeks to answer these and related questions through an examination of the practice of a range of international tribunals concerned with allegations of torture.

International tribunals which examine allegations of torture may be either criminal or civil in nature. The basic separator in the following discussions will be the distinction between tribunals which deal with cases of individual criminal responsibility (international criminal tribunals), and those which are responsible for determining the primarily civil responsibility of States (human rights tribunals). As the focus is on international tribunals, the decisions of which are legally binding or at least declaratory of a violation of international obligations, non-judicial and national fora will not be considered.

International criminal tribunals have been relatively few and far between, and practice is limited to that of the post-World War 2 war crimes tribunals at Nuremberg and Tokyo and the two *ad hoc* tribunals for the former Yugoslavia and Rwanda, as well as related rules of procedure and evidence including those of the imminent International Criminal Court (ICC). Human rights tribunals, on the other hand, have a well-developed jurisprudence which permits a much greater specificity of analysis. In particular, the case-law of the European Court and Commission on Human Rights and of the Inter-American Court and Commission on Human Rights has been valuable in attempting to extract principles concerning their approach to medical evidence, with additional practice also relied on from the UN Human Rights Committee and the UN Committee Against Torture (CAT).

GENERAL RULES RELATING TO EVIDENCE BEFORE INTERNATIONAL TRIBUNALS

The role of medical evidence cannot meaningfully be discussed without first identifying the general rules on burden and standard of proof, as well as the evaluation of evidence, which operate in the context of international tribunals. These rules and practices are applicable to medical evidence in the same way as to any other form of evidence. The tribunals have been uniformly adamant that their approach to evidence is a flexible one, with the implication that there are no fixed rules with respect to medical evidence. How has this been borne out in practice?

A preliminary question is to ask if international tribunals can take a proactive approach to evidence. This requires consideration of the relationship between international tribunals and their domestic counterparts. Can they exercise an independent fact-finding role or must they be bound by the findings of domestic courts where an investigation has taken place? What happens where there has been no domestic investigation?

As a rule, it is up to the party who is attempting to establish the responsibility of the other party to provide convincing evidence to substantiate their claim – that party bears the burden of proof. Under certain conditions, that burden may be reversed, so that the burden is on the accused party to show that they are not responsible. What might those conditions be, and does medical evidence have a particular part to play in such a reversal of the burden of proof? The party bearing the burden of proof must also discharge that burden to a certain standard, which varies according to the nature of the proceedings.

The differing nature of the two types of tribunals has particular implications for burden and standard of proof. On the one hand, international criminal tribunals require a high standard of proof, because it must be established that the accused is guilty of a crime. On the other hand, not only does guilt not have to be proven in order for a State to be held responsible for a violation under human rights law, but also the special conditions of operation give rise to problems with the reliability of evidence. Allegations of human rights violations have an undeniable political dimension, and intimidation and reprisals are common official responses to such allegations.[2] How have human rights tribunals attempted to address such difficulties in developing their approach to evidence?

Further issues arise in relation to the individual pieces of evidence themselves. First, they should fulfil certain basic criteria in order to be admitted by the tribunal. If they are admissible, an assessment of the weight to be attributed to them, their probative value, must then be made. Have the international tribunals developed any distinct rules in this respect? It should also be asked if a single piece of evidence can ever provide a sufficient basis for a finding of responsibility or if corroboration is a requirement.

International criminal tribunals

Relationship with the national system

The Rules of Procedure and Evidence for international criminal tribunals tend not to be particularly precise with respect to the admissibility and evaluation of evidence. This is true both of the *ad hoc* tribunals and of the newly adopted rules for the ICC. What is consistent, however, is for these tribunals to assert their independence from national systems, stating that they are neither bound by national rules of evidence, nor required to apply any particular legal system.[3] Their approach is instead a flexible one, choosing to admit and evaluate evidence 'in a manner best favoured to a fair determination of the matter, consonant with the spirit of the statute and the general principles of international law'.[4]

Burden of proof

The principal burden of proof, as with any criminal case, is on the Prosecution to demonstrate the guilt of the Accused.[5] Where the Defence wishes to make a claim in response to a piece of evidence submitted by the Prosecution, the burden is on it to provide supporting evidence for that claim. Specifically in relation to crimes of sexual violence, the International Criminal Tribunal for Rwanda (ICTR) has stated that where first-hand accounts of sexual violence have been provided, it is not sufficient for the Defence merely to deny the charges without also submitting evidence in support of the claim of fabrication.[6] A similar burden exists on the Defence if it wishes to claim that a witness has supplied false testimony – it cannot merely cast doubts on the credibility of the statements, but must also establish a wilful intent to provide false testimony.[7]

Standard of proof

As is generally the case for criminal proceedings in countries with a commonwealth legal tradition, the standard of proof with respect to establishing that the acts in question were committed by the Accused is proof beyond reasonable doubt.[8] As will be seen below, this same test is also adopted by the European Court of Human Rights in civil proceedings relating to state responsibility.

Admissibility of evidence

The international criminal tribunals take a broad approach to admissibility rather than formulating a set of technical rules.[9] The determining factor in deciding to take evidence into account is probative value. In the context of the Nuremberg trials, evidence could be admitted if it appeared authentic and was deemed of probative value.[10] Similarly, the two *ad hoc* tribunals may admit any evidence which is both relevant and considered to have probative value.[11] The ICTR elaborates that reliability is a factor in finding evidence to be relevant and of probative value, but not a separate head of admissibility. Reliability should also not be equated with credibility, and evidence which is found to be reliable for the purposes of admissibility may later be found not credible. The burden of proof in establishing admissibility is on the party wishing to rely on the evidence. The evidence must be shown to have some relevance and some probative value, on the balance of probabilities.[12] Evidence may be excluded if its probative value is deemed to be substantially outweighed by the need to ensure a fair trial,[13] or if it was obtained in a way which casts substantial doubt on its reliability or its admission would damage the integrity of the proceedings.[14]

Corroboration

Corroboration is not required as a matter of law before the international criminal tribunals. This is affirmed in the rules and practice of both *ad hoc* tribunals,[15] and repeated in the ICC Rules of Procedure and Evidence.[16] The *ad hoc* tribunals have firmly rejected the argument that this applies only to crimes of sexual violence.[17]

The recently adopted ICC rules have built on this experience of the *ad hoc* tribunals by expressly excluding such an interpretation, stating that corroboration is not legally required to prove *any* crime before the ICC. Consequently, the testimony of a single witness may be relied on, provided the witness appears reliable and the evidence credible, a matter for the tribunal to consider.[18] In particular, in response to Defence arguments that allegations of ill-treatment were not supported by medical evidence, and thus not objectively established, both the Trial and Appeal Chambers of the International Criminal Tribunal for the former Yugoslavia (ICTY) stated that medical reports or other scientific evidence were not required as proof of a material fact, and that evidence could be given by other means provided it was sufficient to satisfy the tribunal beyond reasonable doubt that the acts of violence had been committed.[19]

Corroboration is, nonetheless, an important factor in evaluating the probative value of evidence. Evidence which is supported by other evidence will be viewed as having greater probative value, unless neither piece of evidence is considered credible. In particular, oral testimony may be used to corroborate written evidence – for example, the author of a medical report may give evidence in person before the tribunal explaining and confirming his or her findings. Independent evidence can be used to prove or disprove the probative value of a piece of documentary evidence, as long as that independent evidence is also admissible. While corroboration may increase the probative value of a piece of evidence, it is not determinative, and does not establish absolute credibility. [20]

Probative value

The probative value of a piece of evidence is attributed on the basis of its credibility and relevance to the allegations being made. It should be assessed in the context of all other evidence presented. The ICTR has identified three factors in assessing the credibility of a piece of documentary evidence.[21] The first is the relationship between the document and its source. It considers it inappropriate to automatically disallow evidence which emanates from the person seeking to rely on it, unless the particular piece of evidence is deemed irrelevant or of no probative value, but the source may nonetheless affect the assessment of reliability or credibility.

The next factor is the authenticity of the document and its contents. In assessing this, the tribunal may take into account such matters as the form, contents and purported use of the document. For example, an original document will generally have a higher probative value than a copy, as will a document marked with an official stamp or other form of certification. The tribunal will normally seek to rely on more than one such factor in determining authenticity and may request verification, including through expert testimony.

In assessing the probative value of a document, the tribunal will also take into account any inconsistencies between the document and oral testimony. The weight given to such discrepancies will depend on the circumstances in which the prior statement was made and that statement's reliability and credibility. In principle, most weight will be given to prior statements made before a judicial body, but conflicting evidence under oath needs to be addressed on a case by case basis, examining in particular any explanations given by the witness for the inconsistencies.

Human rights tribunals

Relationship with the national system

As with international criminal tribunals, human rights tribunals are not bound to apply domestic legal procedures and have instead developed their own approaches to evidence.[22] The central issue is the extent to which such tribunals are entitled to make their own findings of fact. There is general agreement among the tribunals that they may make such evaluations, but not always with equal enthusiasm.

The Inter-American Court of Human Rights takes the approach that its power to weigh evidence freely is recognised in international jurisprudence, reserving the right to adopt a flexible approach to the amount of proof necessary to support its conclusions.[23]

The European Court of Human Rights and its former Commission, while acknowledging that it is not in principle their task to substitute their own assessment of the facts for those of the domestic courts, have consistently affirmed that they are not bound by the findings of the domestic courts.[24] In order to depart from the findings of those courts, an examination must be made of all the materials submitted, with a view to identifying any 'cogent elements which could call into question the findings of the national court and add weight to the applicant's allegations'.[25] In the absence of such elements, the Court has generally accepted the domestic findings of fact, even where the Commission had previously found the allegations plausible,[26] but this should not be taken as an indication that domestic findings of fact are accepted as reliable as a matter of course. A mere reference by the defendant State to the findings of domestic proceedings is not considered sufficient to cast doubt on the account of a victim.[27]

The Human Rights Committee takes the view that it is in principle not for it to question the evaluation of evidence made by national courts and, while retaining the authority to do so, adopts more restrictive criteria than the two regional courts, stating that it will do so where the findings are 'manifestly arbitrary or constituting a denial of justice'.[28]

Burden of proof

The burden of proof in proceedings before human rights tribunals originates in the special nature of those proceedings. This has two aspects. First, responsibility under an international human rights treaty is unlike responsibility of individuals for criminal offences. Its aim is to provide redress for the victim and does not require any guilt on the part of the State.[29] The second aspect is that access to evidence is not equal between the two parties – the State 'controls the means to verify acts occurring within its territory'.[30] These factors have led the international tribunals to adopt a number of presumptions and a reversal of the burden of proof in certain circumstances.

The Regulations of the Inter-American Commission on Human Rights allow it to presume the facts of a petition to be true if the government fails to respond or to provide pertinent information once the petition has been transmitted to it.[31] The Commission elaborates in its case-law that it is not the mere failure on the part of the State to supply information which makes the facts true. The petition must contain sufficient information for it to be admissible, and it must be consistent, credible and specific enough to enable the Commission to evaluate the facts. If these conditions are satisfied, then 'silence, or elusive or ambiguous answers on the part of the State may be interpreted as an acknowledgement of the truth of the allegations'.[32] A similar approach is adopted by the Human Rights Committee.[33]

In both regional systems, once *prima facie* evidence has been presented, the burden of proof is on the State to show that it investigated the allegation and that physical violence did not occur.[34] This is particularly true where persons are in state custody, whether police custody or prison,[35] and thus under the exclusive control of the State.[36] In such cases, where an individual was in good health upon entering custody and injuries are subsequently found on his or her body, the government is required to provide a plausible explanation of how the injuries were caused, and to produce evidence which casts doubt on the account of the victim.[37] It is not sufficient for the government merely to offer an explanation in order for the burden to be met – if the reasons provided are found not to convincingly explain the injuries reported, the presumption will not be considered rebutted.[38] The presumption in favour of the claimant is at its strongest in cases of disappearance.[39]

Standard of proof

Under the European Convention on Human Rights, the standard of proof adopted when evaluating evidence in relation to an allegation of ill-treatment is that of 'beyond reasonable doubt'. Such proof may follow 'from the coexistence of sufficiently strong, clear and concordant inferences or of similar unrebutted presumptions of fact'.[40] The Commission goes on to specify that a reasonable doubt means 'not a doubt based merely on a theoretical possibility, but a doubt for which reasons can be drawn from the facts presented'. Where injuries have occurred during custody, it is not sufficient for the government to point at other possible causes in order to cast a doubt on the victim's account. Instead it is required to produce evidence showing facts which cast such a doubt.[41] The Inter-American Commission on Human Rights further specifies that where the State fails to provide information and the facts are well-founded, the petitioner should not be expected to satisfy the same standard of proof as if the State had responded.[42]

Admissibility

The Rules of the Inter-American Court of Human Rights specify that the Court may obtain 'any evidence it considers helpful' and may invite the parties to provide any evidence that in its opinion 'may be useful'.[43] The Court states that 'the practice of international and domestic courts shows that direct evidence, whether testimonial or documentary, is not the only type of evidence that may be legitimately considered. Circumstantial evidence, indicia and presumptions may be considered so long as they lead to conclusions consistent with the facts', particularly in cases of disappearance.[44] The Rules of the European Court of Human Rights do not expressly address the question of admissibility of evidence, but do provide for the taking of evidence, either at the request of the parties or on the Court's own initiative.[45]

THE ROLE OF MEDICAL EVIDENCE BEFORE INTERNATIONAL TRIBUNALS

Turning to the role of medical evidence in particular, the first issue is to consider what effect, if any, such evidence may have on the burden of proof. The central question, following on from this, is whether it is ever the determining factor in a tribunal finding or if other elements must always be present. Might this depend on the nature of the medical evidence or the objective pursued? Might it depend on the availability of other items of evidence, either medical or non-medical in nature?

International criminal tribunals

Identifying specific principles and criteria in relation to medical evidence is difficult in the context of the international criminal tribunals which have operated until now. As a rule, these tribunals have focused on bringing to justice those they term the 'big fish' or whose violations may be qualified as flagrant. The evidence in such cases tends to be overwhelming and not, therefore, addressed individually in the judgment,[46] or much of the discussion centres on matters of principle.[47] What clearly emerges, however, is that medical evidence is not a requirement for an allegation of torture to be considered proven. The ICTR states that 'the absence of forensic or real evidence shall in no way diminish the probative value of evidence provided; in particular, the absence of forensic evidence corroborating eyewitness testimonies shall in no way affect the assessment of those testimonies'.[48] On occasions when the Defence has submitted arguments to the contrary, the tribunal has either failed to address them [49] or firmly rejected them, including on appeal.[50]

Human rights tribunals

Medical evidence is most likely to be an issue in connection with its submission by the claimant. The State may, however, also seek to submit its own contradictory evidence, or may be expected to do so in support of its defence. In order to attempt to evaluate the role played by medical evidence, it is necessary to consider cases in which ill-treatment has been alleged without the support of medical evidence, on the one hand, and those cases where medical evidence has been provided, on the other. The role of medical evidence submitted by the State is considered separately.

If there is no medical evidence

The human rights tribunals appear to have been very careful not to make medical evidence a requirement for those seeking to establish that ill-treatment has occurred. The European Court of Human Rights has expressly recognised that medical evidence was unlikely to be available in cases of unacknowledged detention and disappearance, and considered that to require it as a prerequisite for a finding of violation of the article prohibiting torture 'would undermine the protection offered by that provision'.[51] Each of the tribunals has regularly found facts proved beyond reasonable doubt in the absence of medical evidence.[52] When they have not done so, they have tended to refer to other factors in reaching their decision, such as an unexplained failure to bring the allegations to the attention of lawyers at an early stage,[53] or a failure to provide explanations for inconsistencies in the accounts given to the authorities at different times.[54] Other forms of evidence which have contributed to the establishment of facts in the absence of medical evidence include victim and witness statements,[55] a piece of cloth used as a blindfold during the ill-treatment, and photographs.[56] Alternative forms of evidence aside, two factors appear to have played a significant role in the decisions of the tribunals: the extent to which the allegations have been investigated at the domestic level, and the degree of specificity of the allegation.

Where an allegation has been satisfactorily investigated at the domestic level, and no medical evidence has been submitted in support of the allegation, the tribunals have tended to find the allegation unproven.[57] This distinction is particularly noteworthy where, in the same case, one alleged form of ill-treatment which had not been established by the domestic courts and was not supported by medical evidence was found not to have been established, while other ill-treatment of the same individual was supported by medical certificates and found to constitute torture.[58] In contrast, where precise details were provided and no effective investigation appeared to have been carried out, the tribunals tended to find the facts established even in the absence of medical evidence.[59] Furthermore, with respect to the specificity of the allegation, while detailed allegations have been accepted quite willingly by the tribunals, generally-phrased [60] or skeletal accusations have more often been rejected – for example, the Inter-American Commission on Human Rights considered it insufficient to make reference to an injury without providing any further description or evidence of the injury or its cause.[61]

If there is medical evidence

Does it prima facie affect the burden of proof?

In addition to the presumptions and reversal of burden of proof previously discussed in general terms, such a transference of the burden of proof to the government has often been imposed specifically where an allegation was considered substantiated through reliance on medical reports.[62] In particular, this presumption has operated where the medical reports provided evidence that injuries had occurred during a period of detention and the government was unable to provide a plausible explanation for them.[63] The European Court of Human Rights has also referred to the medical reports which created the presumption in order to dismiss the explanations offered by the government as unconvincing.[64] The CAT on one occasion found a State party in breach of its obligation of *non-refoulement* where it failed to provide an explanation as to why it did not consider two medical reports indicating psychological difficulties as sufficiently substantial to warrant a medical examination under its procedures for asylum applications.[65]

Is it sufficient for a finding of violation?

In order to assess the exact role of medical evidence in a finding of violation, it is necessary to ask if such evidence is ever sufficient to make such a finding, and what factors are taken into account in such findings. Three considerations may be identified as especially influential in assessing the role of a particular piece of medical evidence. First, for what purpose is the evidence being submitted? Is the overall aim to establish a direct violation for the acts in question, an indirect violation, for example, for failure to investigate, or a previous incident of torture for the purposes of preventing an expulsion? The question in this case is whether or not medical evidence plays a different role according to the objective for which it is submitted. Secondly, what does the content of the evidence show? Does it testify merely to the presence of injuries, or also to causality between the injuries or state of mind of the person and the treatment alleged? Finally, with what degree of certainty, or how conclusively, does the evidence set out its findings?

Relevant cases may be divided into two broad categories: those which seek to establish that the State is responsible for an incident of torture and those which attempt to prevent the expulsion of an individual to a country where he or she is believed to be at risk of torture. The distinction is important because it appears to affect the attitude adopted by the tribunals to medical evidence.

Responsibility for an incident of ill-treatment

In cases seeking to establish the responsibility of a State for an incident of ill-treatment, the exact role of medical evidence revolves around the related issues of causality and certainty or, more precisely, the degree of certainty with which causality may be demonstrated. If causality can be established with some degree of certainty, a direct violation may be found. Even where the findings are insufficiently conclusive for a direct violation, the State may still be found responsible for an indirect violation.

Establishing causality with a sufficient degree of certainty should, where possible, rely on two components: the injuries should be shown to be consistent with the treatment alleged, and other possible causes for the injuries should be excluded. For example, where medical evidence showed that the victim suffered from bilateral radial paralysis, the analysis of the European Commission on Human Rights focused on the question of whether or not it could have had another cause than the treatment alleged. It concluded on the basis of the medical evidence that although radial paralysis had other possible causes, a bilateral occurrence of such paralysis was rare and most consistent with Palestinian hanging, a form of suspension by the arms. In the absence of an explanation from the Government, it was found established that the victim had been tortured while in custody.[66] The Court has recently endorsed the comments of the European Committee for the Prevention of Torture that a medical report must include not only details of the injuries found, but also the explanations provided by the patient as to how they occurred and the opinion of the doctor as to whether the injuries are consistent with those explanations.[67]

The degree of certainty with which tribunals have required causality to be demonstrated in order to make a finding of violation has not always been consistent and, as a general rule, where causality has been less certain, the tribunals have in any case taken other factors into account in reaching their decision. The most persuasive evidence has consisted of 'precise and concurring medical evidence', several medical reports which are mutually reinforcing and track the condition of the victim over a period of time. Such evidence has been considered particularly compelling in a custodial context.[68] Individual pieces of evidence which have been relied on to find that a violation had occurred include statements that injuries 'could only have been' or were 'irrefutably' caused by the treatment alleged,[69] were 'consistent with' that treatment,[70] or 'not inconsistent with' it.[71] In one case in which a violation was found where the medical evidence relied on was considered 'not inconsistent with' the injuries, conflicting government evidence also existed which gave no explanation for using a dating technique different to that most commonly accepted, and the applicant and her father were considered credible witnesses.[72] Evidence which was accepted as substantiating a complaint of torture includes a psychiatric report showing that the applicant was suffering from post-traumatic stress disorder (PTSD) consistent with the torture alleged.[73] Where evidence was considered inconclusive or unconvincing, no violation has been found.[74]

The lesser the degree of certainty, the more importance is placed on accompanying factors. Where the medical evidence establishes the presence of injuries but does not suggest a cause, the tribunals have made findings of both violation and non-violation. For example, no violation was found in one case where the description of events was considered vague and no information was provided about the manner of the ill-treatment.[75] In another case, a violation was found even though it was not possible to establish a causal link, where the Court considered that the surrounding factors (the victim's testimony, the fact that he had been detained at the police station for two hours, failure of witness accounts to support an alternative explanation for the injuries) were sufficient to establish a reasonable suspicion that the injuries might have been caused by the police.[76] In this case, the violation was an indirect one, for failure to investigate the incident.

Two further conclusions may be drawn from the jurisprudence. The first is that establishing causality with any degree of certainty is less determinative where injuries have been suffered in custody. In such a case, where the medical evidence sets out both the presence of injuries and the probable date of their occurrence, coinciding with the period of custody, this has been found to reverse the burden of proof, and has been relied on to find the State responsible at least for an indirect violation.[77] Where it is not possible to prove that the alleged victim was in custody, the extent to which causality can be conclusively established becomes more important. It is not sufficient, for example, to point to a medical report showing bruising,[78] although additional factors may still lead the tribunal to find that an indirect violation has occurred.[79]

The second conclusion is that, where the medical evidence does not establish causality with a sufficient degree of certainty to prove a direct violation beyond reasonable doubt, the tribunals have tended to fall back on a finding of indirect violation, for failure to conduct an effective investigation or to protect the right to physical integrity, and have done so with increasing frequency in recent cases.[80] In one case involving a dead body showing marks of ill-treatment, it was considered established that the victim had been in captivity, and thus that the State had failed to protect his right to life and to physical integrity, even though the circumstances of the treatment and death were unknown.[81] In cases where injuries were reported in the medical evidence but no causal link was established, the Court found that an investigation ought to have taken place, even where little detail was provided about the form of the treatment.[82] Where no causal link was established and the victim was in custody for only part of the time during which the injuries might have been caused, the Court found that enough factors existed to give rise to a reasonable suspicion that the police might be responsible, and thus that the matter ought to have been investigated.[83]

Expulsion

In expulsion cases, the claimant is not trying to establish that the State has been implicated in an incident of torture. Instead, the person is seeking to invoke a previous incident of torture as a factor to be taken into account by the tribunal when deciding if a risk exists that he or she will be tortured if returned. This essentially goes to the credibility of the claim, and the tribunals appear to have adopted a less stringent approach in determining the degree of certainty of causality required than in the case of direct State responsibility for an occurrence of ill-treatment. Although it has been established with a high degree of certainty in certain cases,[84] such a threshold has not been a requirement and, at best, the test may be on the balance of probabilities. Previous incidents of torture have been considered established where the evidence stated that the scars 'could only have been caused by' the treatment alleged[85] or 'could have been caused by' it,[86] and where the evidence was 'consistent with' the allegation,[87] or '(did) not contradict' it.[88] The tribunals have shown themselves very willing to accept evidence of PTSD as a convincing step in establishing previous torture,[89] unless that evidence is presented without actually claiming that torture has occurred, as happened in one instance.[90] In particular, they have considered PTSD to excuse many inconsistencies in a victim's account, on the ground that accuracy should not normally be expected from a victim of torture. The issue in these cases is the establishment of current risk, and this is what the tribunals have focused on. Although they have been flexible in concluding that an individual has been tortured in the past, they will still seek to establish that the risk of torture is a current one, failing which the deportation may proceed.[91]

Its relationship with other items of evidence or factors

As may be expected, the tribunals have tended to base their reasoning in any particular case on the body of evidence taken as a whole. This makes it difficult to isolate the relationship of a specific piece of medical evidence with other pieces of evidence, whether medical or non-medical in nature. The tribunals often refer to evidence which above all helps to reinforce the credibility of the allegation. The existence of supporting medical evidence, either confirming the findings of the piece of medical evidence in question or dismissing the plausibility of the official explanations, appears particularly persuasive. Conflicting medical evidence submitted by the State has, in general, been approached with caution.

Factors which have been taken into account in combination with medical evidence submitted by the claimant in making a finding of violation or potential violation include family background, political activities, and indications that the person is presently wanted in the country to which he or she is about to be returned (for a finding under Article 3 of the UN Convention Against Torture);[92] statements by witnesses convinced of the correctness of the applicant's account, an independent medical opinion and forensic report that the police account was implausible, and a statement that a footprint was visible on clothing at the site of an injury;[93] the incomplete nature of the state autopsy examination and the unreliable nature of police evidence.[94] Factors taken into account when deciding that medical certificates did not support the allegations include a lack of detailed account of the abuse, the fact that the applicant was never refused permission to see a doctor, the fact that the applicant had made several complaints through his lawyer but not about these particular allegations, and the fact that no complaint was made until a year after the ill-treatment stopped, without offering an explanation for the delay. In that case, however, a violation was found on the ground of lack of an effective investigation.[95]

Where significant conflicting medical evidence has been submitted by both parties, there appears to be a tendency to find in favour of the complainant on some other ground. In one case, where major disparities in the findings of forensic officials as to the causes of some of the injuries could have been resolved by exhuming the body, the CAT interpreted the failure of the State to do so as a failure to investigate thoroughly and impartially.[96] When presented with conflicting medical evidence in a disappearance case in which bodies had been found, the Inter-American Commission on Human Rights considered the facts as a whole, preferred the petitioner's evidence to that of the government and concluded that the allegations were true.[97] Nor has the European Commission on Human Rights been convinced by governmental medical evidence relying on approaches to the dating of injuries which differ from those generally accepted, where no explanation has been provided for such a divergence.[98]

The role of State medical evidence

Burden of proof

Is there ever an obligation on the State to provide medical evidence? There is some indication that it would not be sufficient for the State to deny the existence of severe injury without submitting medical evidence in support of its claim.[99] Similarly, where a State wishes to refer to the findings of a domestic investigation contested by the complainant, it would not be sufficient for it merely to refer without providing copies of the reports, especially where the explanations for the injuries are considered unconvincing by the tribunal.[100] In another case, where the State submitted medical evidence that an injury predated the alleged incidents, the CAT requested the State to obtain a further examination by an independent expert.[101]

Probative value

The tribunals appear to have adopted a distinctly sceptical approach to State medical evidence in general, and have tended to find the evidence unconvincing, or else not inconsistent with the allegations. In one case, the evidence of a petitioner who saw the body was found more convincing than a State medical–legal report identifying the cause of death as cardiac arrest.[102] In another, although the government supplied X-rays indicating that a claimant's jaw was not broken in spite of her allegation that it had been, the European Commission on Human Rights remained convinced of the credibility of the applicant and of her account.[103] The Court similarly considered that medical evidence which suggested hypothetical causes for an injury, without indicating why this was more probable than the applicant's account, could not be relied on to rebut the applicant's allegation of rape in custody.[104] Most recently, the Court has endorsed the statement of the European Committee for the Prevention of Torture that proper medical examinations of persons in custody must be 'carried out by a properly qualified doctor, without any police officer being present and the report of the examination must include not only the detail of any injuries found but the explanations given by the patient as to how they occurred and the opinion of the doctor as to whether the injuries are consistent with those explanations'.[105] Where a State submitted medical evidence showing no signs of injuries or scars, the Inter-American Commission on Human Rights countered that the right to personal integrity encompasses more than a ban on beatings, physical torture or other forms of treatment that leaves visible marks on the victim,[106] and also considered in another case that such a certificate was not inconsistent with the allegations where it had not been carried out until one year after the incident, when it would be unlikely to find physical signs of mistreatment.[107]

Approach to inadequacy or absence of State medical evidence

The tribunals have shown a tendency to rely on the inadequacy or absence of State medical evidence in order to make a finding of failure to investigate. In one case where there was disagreement between experts as to the dating of bruises, the CAT found that the time elapsed between the report of bruising and action by the judge was incompatible with the obligation for a prompt investigation, and that other evidence ought to have been called as forensic medical reports are important but often insufficient.[108] In another case, the European Commission on Human Rights was of the opinion that the lack of a timely investigation made it impossible to resolve conflicting accounts of events, and that the issuing of a medical certificate two days after the incident in question made it impossible to establish causality. The Court in this case found that the bruising referred to in the certificate ought nonetheless to have sparked off an investigation, and found a violation on this basis.[109] Similarly, the Court found that even where it was not possible to establish that injuries were caused by the police, the presence of fresh bruising ought to have prompted an investigation, in the absence of which there had been a violation.[110] Both the Human Rights Committee and the Inter-American Commission on Human Rights have relied on the deficiency of State medical evidence as a factor in finding that investigation had been inadequate.[111]

CONCLUSIONS

International tribunals, whether criminal in nature or concerned with human rights, have affirmed that they are not bound by national rules of evidence. They are also free to make their own findings of fact, particularly where those of the domestic courts have been called into question. The burden of proof for establishing responsibility for the acts in question before both kinds of tribunals lies initially with the party making the allegation, but the approach of human rights tribunals to the burden of proof has evolved in response to the particularly sensitive nature of human rights claims. Where *prima facie* evidence is presented in support of a claim of violation, the burden of proof may shift to the State to show that it investigated and that the acts did not happen or that an effective remedy was provided. If the State is silent and the evidence presented is considered consistent, credible and specific, the facts may be presumed to be true, at least under the Inter-American system and before the Human Rights Committee. Such presumptions are particularly strong where it is established that the victim was in custody when he or she received the injuries. The standard of proof adopted before international criminal tribunals is that of 'beyond reasonable doubt'. This is also the standard adopted by the regional human rights tribunals, even though proceedings before them are essentially civil in nature.

Both types of tribunals have adopted a flexible approach to the admissibility of evidence, with very broad formulations. International criminal tribunals specify that evidence should be relevant and of probative value, as well as reliable, while human rights tribunals will consider any evidence they consider helpful or pertinent to the case. Corroboration is not required as a matter of law in either context, but it is an important factor in evaluating the probative value of any piece of evidence. Probative value before the international tribunals is attributed on the basis of credibility and relevance to the allegation being made, and should be assessed in the context of all other evidence presented.

International criminal tribunals have not as yet provided precise discussions on the role of medical evidence in their public judgments, but they have made it clear that it is not a requirement for an allegation of torture to be considered proven, and that its absence does not reduce the probative value of other evidence.

The jurisprudence of human rights tribunals similarly reveals that medical evidence is not a prerequisite for a finding of violation of the prohibition of torture and inhuman treatment, but that it is very persuasive. In the absence of medical evidence, although findings of violation have been made, it is crucial to strengthen the case in other ways, in particular by ensuring that the allegations are as detailed as possible.

In order for it to be of consequence, medical evidence should, as a minimum, establish the presence of injuries or of symptoms of some psychological disorder. Ideally, it should indicate not only the details of the injuries or disorder, but also report the alleged causes of the injuries and comment on the extent to which the injuries are consistent with the treatment alleged. In addition, where possible, it should seek to exclude other possible causes of the injuries.

Medical evidence which indicates the presence of injuries may suffice to create a presumption that the allegations are true in the absence of a plausible explanation by the government in question. This is particularly true where the injuries can be reliably dated as having occurred during a period of custody, and most compelling when the injuries can be shown to have appeared and developed over the period in question in a series of medical reports. In such cases, the medical evidence may be sufficient for a finding of at least an indirect violation. As a general rule, the role of medical evidence is less determinative than this in the sense that it will be considered in the context of the evidence as a whole. Nonetheless, it may be reliably concluded that medical evidence which indicates that injuries have been received, and that those injuries are consistent with the ill-treatment alleged, excluding where possible alternative causes for the injuries, will be given significant weight in the decision of the tribunal.

A somewhat less stringent approach to medical evidence has been demonstrated in cases involving the proposed expulsion of a person to a country where he or she is alleged to be at risk of torture. This may be explained by the fact that the objective in such cases is to assess the current risk to the person and evidence of previous torture is merely a factor in making this assessment rather than seeking to support the attribution of responsibility for the ill-treatment.

Medical evidence supplied by the State has generally been approached with caution and has even been relied on by the human rights tribunals to support a finding of inadequate investigation where it was considered deficient or inconclusive.

Although many evidential questions have not yet been answered conclusively, or perhaps even addressed, by the existing body of jurisprudence, some tendencies have nonetheless begun to emerge. Some are common to both types of international tribunals, while others have developed in the context of either one or the other. This is not to suggest, however, that some cross-fertilisation might not be appropriate. At this stage, the practice of the human rights tribunals is a great deal more enlightening on the question of medical evidence than that of the criminal tribunals. Although the nature of the proceedings is different, and a very distinct approach to the burden of proof has been adopted by the human rights tribunals, the standard of proof adopted in each case is the same, that of 'beyond reasonable doubt'. The application of that standard in State responsibility cases, the purpose of which is to provide a victim with a remedy, may be less stringent than in individual criminal cases, the consequences of which are penal. Nonetheless, it may well be that many of the principles sketched out in the practice of the human rights tribunals could lend themselves to some application before the international criminal tribunals.

REFERENCES

1 Sections VI–VII and Appendices I–IV, Manual on the Effective Investigation and Documentation of Torture and other Cruel, Inhuman or Degrading Treatment or Punishment (Istanbul Protocol) (see: Welsh J. The problem of torture, Chapter 1 in this book)
2 See, e.g., Ergi v. Turkey (Application No. 23818/94), Judgment of the European Court of Human Rights of 28 July 1998, para. 105; Akkoc v. Turkey (Application No. 22947/93; 22948/93), Judgment of the European Court of Human Rights of 10 October 2000, paras 120–127; Tanrikulu v. Turkey (Application No. 23763/94), Judgment of the European Court of Human Rights of 8 July 1999, paras 126–133; Cabellero Delgado and Santana Case, Provisional Measures requested by the Inter-American Commission of Human Rights regarding Colombia, 7 December 1994; Carpio Nicolle Case, Provisional Measures in the Matter of Guatemala, Order of the Court of 10 September 1996; Decision of the Inter-American Court of Human Rights, 27 January 1993, Provisional Measures requested by the Inter-American Commission of Human Rights regarding Peru, Chipoco Case. All judgments and rules of the Inter-American Court of Human Rights and reports and regulations of the Inter-American Commission of Human Rights referred to in this

chapter may be found at http://www1.umn.edu/humanrts/iachr/iachr.htm. All judgments and rules of the European Court of Human Rights and reports of the European Commission on Human Rights referred to in this chapter may be found at http://www.echr.coe.int

3 Rules of Procedure and Evidence of the International Criminal Court, UN Doc. PCNICC/2000/INF/3/Add. 1, 12 July 2000, Rule 63(4)

4 The Prosecutor v. Georges Rutaganda (ICTR-96-3), Judgment of the Trial Chamber of the International Tribunal for Rwanda, 6 December 1999, para. 17; The Prosecutor v. Jean Paul Akayesu (ICTR-96-4), Judgment of the Trial Chamber of the International Tribunal for Rwanda, 2 September 1998, para. 131; Rules of Procedure and Evidence of the International Criminal Tribunal for Rwanda (ICTR), Consolidated Text as at 26 June 2000, Rule 89(b); Rules of Procedure and Evidence of the International Criminal Tribunal for the Former Yugoslavia (ICTY), Consolidated Text as at 14 July 2000, Rule 89(b), IT/32/Rev. 18. All judgments and rules of the ICTR referred to in this chapter may be found at http://www.ictr.org, and those of the ICTY at http://www.un.org/icty

5 e.g. The Prosecutor v. Anto Furundzija (IT-95-17/1), Judgment of the Trial Chamber of the International Tribunal for the Former Yugoslavia, 10 December 1998, para. 274

6 The Prosecutor v. Akayesu, *supra* note 4, para. 460

7 The Prosecutor v. Georges Rutaganda, *supra* note 4, para. 20; The Prosecutor v. Alfred Musema (ICTR-96-13), Judgment of the Trial Chamber of the International Tribunal for Rwanda, 27 January 2000, para. 99

8 The Prosecutor v. Zlatko Aleksovski (IT-95-14/1), Judgment of the Trial Chamber of the International Tribunal for the Former Yugoslavia, 25 June 1999, para. 223; The Prosecutor v. Anto Furundzija, *supra* note 5, para. 274; The Prosecutor v. Akayesu, *supra* note 4, para. 452

9 Address of Antonio Cassese, President of the ICTY, to the General Assembly of the United Nations, 14 November 1994, reprinted in The 1994 Annual Report of the International Tribunal for the Prosecution of Persons Responsible for Serious Violations of International Humanitarian Law Committed in the Territory of the Former Yugoslavia since 1991, para. 72

10 Regulation 8, Nuremberg Trials Final Report, Appendix E: Royal Warrant – Regulations for the Trial of War Criminals, reproduced at: http://www. yale.edu/lawweb/avalon/images/imtsm.jpg

11 The Prosecutor v. Georges Rutaganda, *supra* note 4, para. 18; The Prosecutor v. Dusko Tadic (IT-94-1), Judgment of the Trial Chamber of the International Tribunal for the Former Yugoslavia, 7 May 1997, para. 536

12 The Prosecutor v. Musema, *supra* note 7, paras 55–58

13 Rules of Procedure and Evidence of the ICTY, *supra* note 4, Rule 89(d)

14 Rules of Procedure and Evidence of the ICTY and ICTR, *supra* note 4, Rule 95

15 Rules of Procedure and Evidence of the ICTY and ICTR, *supra* note 4, Rule 96; The Prosecutor v. Dusko Tadic, see *supra* note 11, para. 536; The Prosecutor v. Georges Rutaganda, *supra* note 4, para.18; The Prosecutor v. Musema, *supra* note 7, paras 43–45; The Prosecutor v. Akayesu, *supra* note 4, paras 134–135

16 Rules of Procedure and Evidence of the International Criminal Court, see *supra* note 3; Rules of Procedure and Evidence of the ICTY and ICTR, *supra* note 4, Rule 96

17 The Prosecutor v. Georges Rutaganda, *supra* note 4, para. 18; The Prosecutor v. Musema, *supra* note 7, para. 45, The Prosecutor v. Akayesu, *supra* note 4, para. 134; The Prosecutor v. Dusko Tadic, see *supra* note 11, para. 536

18 The Prosecutor v. Musema, *supra* note 7, para. 43; The Prosecutor v. Aleksovski (IT-95-14/1), Judgment of the Appeal Chamber of the International Tribunal for the Former Yugoslavia, 24 March 2000, paras 62–63

19 The Prosecutor v. Aleksovski, *supra* note 18, para. 62; The Prosecutor v. Zlatko Aleksovski, *supra* note 8, para. 223

20 The Prosecutor v. Musema, *supra* note 7, paras 46, 75

21 The Prosecutor v. Musema, *supra* note 7, paras 59–97

22 Godínez Cruz Case, Judgment of 20 January 1989, Inter-American Court of Human Rights, (Ser. C) No. 5 (1989), para. 133

23 Godínez Cruz Case, *supra* note 22, paras 133–142

24 e.g. Ribitsch v. Austria (Application No. 18896/91), Report of the European Commission on Human Rights, 4 July 1994, para. 102; Ribitsch v. Austria (Application No. 18896/91), Judgment of the European Court of Human Rights of 4 December 1995, para. 32. The Court has also emphasised that it is not bound by the findings of the European Commission on Human Rights, and that it must make a particularly thorough examination in cases where the findings of the domestic courts and the Commission conflicted, see Ribitsch v. Austria, para. 32; see also Akdivar and Others v. Turkey, Judgment of the European Court of Human Rights of 16 September 1996, para. 78

25 Ribitsch v. Austria, Judgment of the Court, *supra* note 24, para. 32

26 Klaas v. Germany (Application No. 15473/89), Judgment of the European Court of Human Rights of 22 September 1993, para. 30

27 Ribitsch v. Austria, Judgment of the Court, *supra* note 24, para. 34

28 Communication No. 480/1991: Ecuador, 15/08/96, UN Doc. CCPR/C/57/D/480/1991, para. 9.3

29 Anetro Castillo *et al* v. Peru, Cases 10.471, 11.014, 11.067, Report No. 51/99, Inter-American Commission on Human Rights, OEA/Ser.L/V/II.95 Doc. 7 rev. at p 823 (1998), paras 87–92; also Cases 10.544, 10.745, 11.098, Report No. 52/99, Inter-American Commission on Human Rights, OEA/Ser.L/V/II.95 Doc. 7 rev. at p 857 (1998), paras 64–68; Cases 10.807–10, 10.878, 11.307, Report No. 54/99, Inter-American Commission on Human Rights, OEA/Ser.L/V/II.95 Doc. 7 rev. at p 917 (1998), paras 87–92; Cases 10.827, 11.984,

Report No. 57/99, Inter-American Commission on Human Rights, OEA/ Ser.L/V/II.95 Doc. 7 rev. at p 1013 (1998); Godínez Cruz Case, *supra* note 22, para. 140; Ribitsch v. Austria, *supra* note 24

30 Godínez Cruz Case, *supra* note 22, paras 140–142

31 Regulations of the Inter-American Commission on Human Rights, as modified at 3 May 1996, Article 42

32 Raquel Martí de Mejía v. Peru, Case 10.970, Report No. 5/96, Inter-American Commission on Human Rights, OEA/Ser.L/V/II.91 Doc. 7 at p 157 (1996). Factors which contributed to finding information to be sufficiently consistent and specific included the provision of a detailed and consistent version of events, stating the date and place of events, noting the clothing worn and the accompanying soldiers, as well as consistency with commonplace events in the state of emergency area; on the other hand, accounts which did not mention the day or month of the events, provided conflicting versions with disagreement on dates, or mentioned an injury to one victim without providing any further information were found not to fulfil the criteria, see COMADRES v. El Salvador, Case 10.948, Report No. 13/96, Inter-American Commission on Human Rights, OEA/Ser.L/V/II.91 Doc. 7 at p 101 (1996), paras 24.1, 24.2, 24.5, 24.9

33 Communication No. 414/1990: Equatorial Guinea, 10/08/94, UN Doc. CCPR/C/51/D/414/1990, para. 6.2

34 Manuel Garcia Franco v. Ecuador, Case 10.258, Report No. 1/97, Inter-American Commission on Human Rights, OEA/Ser.L/V/II.95 Doc. 7 rev. at p 551 (1997), para. 63

35 Satik and Others v. Turkey (Application No. 31866/96), Judgment of the European Court of Human Rights of 10 October 2000, para. 54

36 Juan Carlos Abella v. Argentina, Case 11.137, Report No. 55/97, Inter-American Commission on Human Rights, OEA/Ser.L/V/II.95 Doc. 7 rev. at p 271 (1997), para. 230

37 Salman v. Turkey (Application No. 21986/93), Judgment of the European Court of Human Rights of 27 June 2000, para. 113; Rehbock v. Slovenia (Application No. 29462/95), Report of the European Commission on Human Rights, 23 April 1999, para. 75; Ribitsch v. Austria, Judgment of the Court, *supra* note 24, para. 34; Aksoy v. Turkey (Application No. 21987/93), Report of the European Commission on Human Rights, 23 October 1995, para. 145; Aksoy v. Turkey (Application No. 22729/93), Judgment of the European Court of Human Rights of 18 December 1996, para. 61; Tomasi v. France (Application No. 12850/87), Judgment of the European Court of Human Rights of 27/08/1992, paras 107–115; Selmouni v. France (Application No. 25803/94), Judgment of the European Court of Human Rights of 28 July 1999, para. 87

38 Satik and Others v. Turkey, *supra* note 35, para. 57. The Government claimed that the injuries in question were caused by a fall down stairs while a group of detainees were linked together. The Court found this to 'sit ill' with the nature

of the injuries noted in the medical reports; Salman v. Turkey (Application No. 21986/93), Report of the European Commission on Human Rights, 1 March 1999. The Government in this case claimed that the victim's fractured sternum had been caused by a resuscitation attempt, but the Commission relied on medical evidence that a fresh bruise overlying the fracture would be unusual in a case of cardiac massage and was more likely the result of trauma. See Sections III C(4) and (5) of the report

39   Anetro Castillo *et al* v. Peru and related cases, *supra* note 29

40   e.g. Ireland v. the United Kingdom (Application No. 05310/71), Judgment of the European Court of Human Rights of 18 January 1978, para. 161; Selmouni v. France (Application No. 25803/94), Judgment of the European Court of Human Rights of 28 July 1999, para. 88; Tekin v. Turkey (Application No. 22496/93), Report of the European Commission on Human Rights, 17 April 1997, para. 171; Kaya v. Turkey (Application No. 22729/93), Report of the European Commission on Human Rights, 24 October 1996, para. 144

41   Ribitsch v. Austria, Report of the Commission, *supra* note 24, para. 104

42   Raquel Martí de Mejía v. Peru, *supra* note 32

43   Rules of Procedure of the Inter-American Court of Human Rights, in effect as of 1 January 1997, Article 44

44   Godínez Cruz Case, *supra* note 18, para. 136; see also Manuel Manriquez v. Mexico, Case 11.509, Report No. 2/99, Inter-American Commission on Human Rights, OEA/Ser.L/V/II.95 Doc. 7 rev. at p 663 (1998), para. 60

45   European Court of Human Rights, Rules of Court as in force at 1 November 1998, Rule 42

46   e.g. Judge Parker, Nuremberg judgment: war crimes and crimes against humanity, reproduced at http://www.yale.edu/lawweb/avalon/images/imtsm.jpg

47   e.g. Much of the discussion in the Tadic Trial Chamber judgment (*supra* note 11) deals with the nature of the conflict

48   The Prosecutor v. Musema, *supra* note 7, para. 52

49   e.g. The Prosecutor v. Akayesu, *supra* note 4, para. 41

50   e.g. The Prosecutor v. Aleksovski, *supra* note 18, paras 57, 62; The Prosecutor v. Zlatko Aleksovski, *supra* note 8, para. 223

51   Cakici v. Turkey (Application No. 23657/94), Judgment of the European Court of Human Rights, 8 July 1999, para. 91, accepting the Commission's opinion on this point

52   Communication No. 598/1994: Jamaica, 25/07/96, UN Doc. CCPR/C/57/D/598/1994; Saravia v. Peru, Case 10.528, Report No. 11/93, Inter-American Commission on Human Rights, OEA/Ser.L/V/II.83 Doc. 14 at p 128 (1993); Manuel Garcia Franco v. Ecuador, *supra* note 34; Victor Hernandez Vasquez v. El Salvador, Case 10.228, Report No. 65/99, Inter-American Commission on Human Rights, OEA/Ser.L/V/II.95 Doc. 7 rev. at p 512 (1998); Tekin v. Turkey, Report of the Commission, *supra* note 40;

Tekin v. Turkey (Application No. 22496/93), Judgment of the European Court of Human Rights of 9 June 1998; Cakici v. Turkey, *supra* note 51

53 Communication No. 649/1995: Jamaica, 25/11/98, UN Doc. CCPR/C/64/D/649/1995, para. 7.3

54 Communication No. 106/1998: Australia, 03/06/99, UN Doc. CAT/C/22/D/106/1998

55 Cakici v. Turkey, *supra* note 51; Saravia v. Peru, *supra* note 52; Manuel Garcia Franco v. Ecuador, *supra* note 34, para. 60–61; Tekin v. Turkey, Report of the Commission, *supra* note 40, paras 188–189; approved by the Court in Tekin v. Turkey, Judgment of the Court, *supra* note 52, paras 48–54

56 Tekin v. Turkey, Report of the Commission, *supra* note 40, para. 190

57 e.g. Communication No. 353/1988: Jamaica, 04/04/94, UN Doc. CCPR/C/50/D/353/1989; Communication No. 6/1990: Spain, 9/06/95, UN Doc. CAT/C/14/D/6/1990

58 Selmouni v. France, *supra* note 37, paras 88–90

59 Communication No. 598/1994: Jamaica, *supra* note 52, para. 8.2; Saravia v. Peru, *supra* note 52

60 Sarközy v. Hungary (Application No. 21967/93), Report of the European Commission on Human Rights, 6 March 1997, para. 84

61 COMADRES v. El Salvador, *supra* note 32, para. 24.9

62 Communication No. 414/1990, *supra* note 33; Klass v. the Federal Republic of Germany (Application No. 15473/89), Report of the European Commission on Human Rights, 21 May 1992, para. 103, although the Court subsequently held that the incident had been satisfactorily investigated by the domestic courts, see Klaas v. Germany, *supra* note 26, para. 30; Ribitsch v. Austria, Report of the Commission, *supra* note 24, affirmed by the Court in Ribitsch v. Austria, Judgment of the Court, *supra* note 24, para. 34

63 Aksoy v. Turkey, Report of the Commission, *supra* note 37, paras 152, 163–164; affirmed by the Court in Aksoy v. Turkey, Judgment of the Court, *supra* note 37, para. 61; Selmouni v. France, *supra* note 37, para. 87

64 Satik and Ors v. Turkey, *supra* note 35, para. 57

65 Communication No. 91/1997: Netherlands, 13/11/98, UN Doc. CAT/C/21/D/91/1997, para. 6.6

66 Aksoy v. Turkey, Report of the Commission, *supra* note 37, paras 164–165; affirmed by the Court in Aksoy v. Turkey, Judgment of the Court, *supra* note 37, para. 61

67 Akkoc v. Turkey, Judgment of the Court, *supra* note 2, para. 118

68 Juan Carlos Abella v. Argentina, *supra* note 36; Selmouni v. France, *supra* note 37; Tomasi v. France, *supra* note 37, paras 107–115

69 Manuel Manriquez v. Mexico, *supra* note 44, para. 49; Chrysostomos and Papachrysostomou v. Turkey (Application No. 15299/89, 15300/89), Report of the European Commission on Human Rights, 8 July 1993, para. 121

70 Communication No. 481/1991: Ecuador, 24/04/97, UN Doc. CCPR/C/ 59/D/481/1991, para. 8.2; Aksoy v. Turkey, Report of the Commission, *supra* note 37, para. 163; affirmed by the Court in Aksoy v. Turkey, Judgment of the Court, *supra* note 37, para. 61

71 Sükran Aydin v. Turkey (Application No. 23178/94), Report of the European Commission on Human Rights, 7 March 1996, paras 163–181

72 Sükran Aydin v. Turkey, *supra* note 71, paras 163–181

73 Akkoc v. Turkey (Application No. 22947-8/93), Report of the European Commission on Human Rights, 23 April 1999, Section III E(1); affirmed by the Court in Akkoc v. Turkey, Judgment of the Court, *supra* note 2

74 Gangaram Panday Case, Judgment of 21 January 1994, Inter-American Court of Human Rights (Ser. C) No. 16 (1994), para. 56

75 Erdagöz v. Turkey (127/1996/945/746), Judgment of the European Court of Human Rights of 22 October 1997, paras 37–43

76 Assenov v. Bulgaria (Application No. 24760/94), Judgment of the European Court of Human Rights of 28 October 1998, paras 101–106

77 Manuel Manriquez v. Mexico, *supra* note 44, paras 49–50; Juan Carlos Abella v. Argentina, *supra* note 36, para. 230; Selmouni v. France, *supra* note 37, para. 87; Tomasi v. France, *supra* note 37, paras 107–115

78 Erdagöz v. Turkey, *supra* note 75, para. 42

79 Assenov v. Bulgaria, Judgment of the Court, *supra* note 76, paras 101–106

80 This emerging pattern of increased reliance by the European Court of Human Rights on findings of indirect violation was noted in a discussion with Professor Malcolm Evans, Professor of Law at the University of Bristol, October 2000

81 Mahmut Kaya v. Turkey (Application No. 22535/93), Report of the European Commission on Human Rights, 23 October 1998, paras 374–375; affirmed in Mahmut Kaya v. Turkey (Application No. 22535/93), Judgment of the European Court of Human Rights of 28 March 2000, paras 110–120

82 Labita v. Italy (Application No. 26772/95), Judgment of the European Court of Human Rights of 6 April 2000; Sevtap Veznedaroglu v. Turkey (Application No. 32357/96), Judgment of the European Court of Human Rights of 11 April 2000, paras 23–35

83 Assenov v. Bulgaria, Judgment of the Court, *supra* note 76, para. 101

84 e.g. Communication No. 43/1996: Sweden, 15/11/96, Annual Report of Committee Against Torture, GAOR 52nd Session, Supplement No. 44 (A/52/44), 10 September 1997, Annex V, para. 10.3; Hatami v. Sweden (Application No. 32448/96), Report of the European Commission on Human Rights, 23 April 1998, para. 104. In both cases, the medical evidence not only affirmed causation but also excluded other possible causes

85 Communication No. 43/1996, *supra* note 84, para. 10.3

86 Communication No. 36/1995: Netherlands, 15/05/96, UN Doc. CAT/C/ 16/D/36/1995, para. 5.4

87 Communication No. 65/1997: Sweden, 06/05/98, UN Doc. CAT/C/20/ D/65/1997; Communication No. 41/1996: Sweden, 13/05/96, UN Doc. CAT/C/16/D/41/1996, para. 3.3; Cruz Varas and Others v. Turkey (Application No. 15576/89), Report of the European Commission on Human Rights, 7 June 1990; Cruz Varas and Others v. Sweden (Application No. 15576/89), Judgment of the European Court of Human Rights of 20 March 1991, para. 77

88 Communication No. 15/1994: Canada, 18/11/94, UN Doc. CAT/C/13/ D/15/1994, para. 12.3

89 e.g. Communication No. 101/1997: Sweden, 16/12/98, UN Doc. CAT/C/ 21/D/101/1997, para. 6.6–6.7; Communication No. 43/1996, *supra* note 84, para. 10.3; Communication No. 41/1996, *supra* note 87, para. 9.3; Communication No. 65/1997, *supra* note 87; Communication No. 96/1997: Netherlands, 24/01/2000, UN Doc. CAT/C/23/D/96/1997

90 Communication No. 38/1995: Switzerland, 09/05/97, UN Doc. CAT/C/18/D/38/1995, para. 10.4

91 e.g. Cruz Varas and Others v. Sweden, Judgment and Commission report, *supra* note 87; Communication No. 36/1995, para. 8, *supra* note 86; Communication No. 65/1997, *supra* note 87

92 Communication No. 101/1997, *supra* note 89, para. 6.7

93 Ribitsch v. Austria, Report of the Commission, *supra* note 24, para. 113; Ribitsch v. Austria, Judgment of the Court, *supra* note 24

94 Salman v. Turkey, Report of the Commission, *supra* note 38, Section C(5) of the report

95 Labita v. Italy, *supra* note 82

96 Communication No. 60/1996: Tunisia, 24/01/2000, UN Doc. CAT/C/23/ D/60/1996, paras 11.9, 11.10, 12

97 Severiano Santiz Gomez *et al* v. Mexico, Case 11.411, Report No. 48/97, Inter-American Commission on Human Rights, OEA/Ser.L/V/II.95 Doc. 7 rev. at p 637 (1997), para. 40

98 Salman v. Turkey, Report of the Commission, *supra* note 38, Section C(5) of the report; Sükran Aydin v. Turkey, *supra* note 71, paras 163–181

99 Communication No. 596/1994: Jamaica, 06/12/95, UN Doc. CCPR/C/55/ D/596/1995, para. 8.2

100 Communications No. 623–624 and 626–627/1995: Georgia, 29/05/98, UN Doc. CCPR/C/62/D/623, 624, 626 and 627/1995, para. 18.6

101 Communication No. 8/1991: Austria, 30/11/93, UN Doc. CAT/C/11/ D/8/1991, para. 10

102 Jose Angel Alas Gomez v. El Salvador, Case 10.190, Report No. 6/92, Inter-American Commission on Human Rights, OEA/Ser.L/V/II.81 Doc. 6 rev.1 at p 99 (1992)

103 Akkoc v. Turkey, Report of the Commission, *supra* note 73, Section III E(1)

104 Aydin v. Turkey (57/1996/676/866), Judgment of the European Court of Human Rights of 25 September 1997, para. 73; Sükran Aydin v. Turkey, *supra* note 71, paras 163–181

105 Akkoc v. Turkey, Judgment of the Court, *supra* note 2, para. 118

106 Loren Laroye Riebe Star *et al* v. Mexico, Case 11.610, Report No. 49/99, Inter-American Commission on Human Rights, OEA/Ser.L/V/II.95 Doc. 7 rev. at p 724 (1998), para. 91

107 Ceferino Ul Musicue and Leolel Coicue v. Colombia, Case 19.853, Report No. 4/98, Inter-American Commission on Human Rights, OEA/Ser.L/V/II.95 Doc. 7 rev. at p 400 (1997), para. 32

108 Communication No. 59/1996: Spain, 14/05/98, UN Doc. CAT/C/20/D/59/1996, para. 8.8

109 Assenov v. Bulgaria (Application No. 24760/94), Report of the European Commission on Human Rights, 10 July 1997, paras 94–96; Assenov v. Bulgaria, Judgment of the Court, *supra* note 76, para. 101

110 Sevtap Veznedaroglu v. Turkey, *supra* note 82, paras 23–35

111 Communication No. 480/1991, *supra* note 28, para. 9.4; Juan Carlos Abella v. Argentina, *supra* note 36

3

DOCUMENTING A WELL-FOUNDED FEAR: HOW MEDICAL CAREGIVERS CAN ASSIST TORTURE SURVIVORS IN THE ASYLUM PROCESS?

Barbara A Frey

INTRODUCTION

In the middle of a busy day at the clinic, a physician enters an examining room to encounter a 30-year-old female patient, recently immigrated from a developing country, who describes consistent and generalized pain. The patient complains of symptoms including headaches, back pain, stomach pain, neck pain, fatigue and joint pain. The patient cannot identify any physical cause for her symptoms and shows obvious reluctance at being examined by the physician. In the twelve minutes scheduled for this general examination, the physician has no chance to delve further into the personal history that might be relevant to the patient's maladies. A week later the physician's office receives a call from a lawyer who asks for the release of the patient's medical records in support of her claim for asylum.

This scenario is taking place on a frequent basis in medical clinics throughout the world. Some medical professionals might have enough knowledge or insight to recognize that an immigrant or refugee patient who presents generalized symptoms like those described above may be a survivor of torture. Other physicians may not have any idea that torture may be a complicating factor in such a patient's history and may even be the underlying etiology of their symptoms.

It is increasingly important for medical caregivers to be aware of the prevalence of torture survivors among their patient population. Not only might a patient's symptoms be related to physical or psychological sequelae from the torture experience, but also without such awareness efforts to treat or heal patients may be misdirected, and medical caregivers may unwittingly subject patients to unnecessary, expensive and painful tests.[1]

The diagnosis and treatment of the torture survivor takes on additional significance when that patient does not have permanent legal residency status in the country where he or she is being treated. The medical records in such a case may be needed to support the patient's claim for asylum, so that the individual and his or her family will not be returned against their will to the place where they were persecuted.

Expert medical and psychological evidence is increasingly necessary for asylum applicants to succeed in their cases. Because of the centrality of the client's credibility to the asylum case, immigration judges and asylum officers frequently request medical and psychological evaluations to corroborate the asylum applicant's story. Many asylum seekers flee their countries of origin under difficult and dangerous circumstances and do not carry with them the kinds of documents that help prove that they were tortured or persecuted. Expert medical testimony can therefore help demonstrate that the applicant's physical and psychological symptoms are consistent with the experiences they describe.[2]

Despite the weight attributed to evidence from health care professionals, there are many barriers to finding appropriate medical and psychological support for asylum applicants. Many immigrants are reluctant to seek out psychological counseling because of the cultural stigma attached to such care.[3] Torture victims may not understand that some of the physical and psychological symptoms they are experiencing can be treated successfully by health care professionals. Torture victims may also fear medical treatment because the clinic or hospital environment may elicit memories of institutionalized ill-treatment or torture. Torture victims who are undocumented immigrants are often reluctant to seek medical treatment because they fear detection by government immigration authorities. Many immigrants lack the money, insurance or access to public benefits that would support health care treatment.[4]

Most asylum applicants do not have the assistance of a lawyer and do not understand what they must prove in order to succeed in their asylum case.[5] Asylum seekers do not have a right to counsel at government expense; they must provide their own attorney or speak for themselves.

When a client is represented by a lawyer, the lawyer may turn to a human rights or refugee organization to help find health care professionals experienced in working with torture victims to examine their client and prepare a medical report.[6] Very few professionals, however, specialize in such care. Lawyers instead must often rely on the records of professionals who may have examined their client during the course of general medical care, much like the scenario described at the beginning of this article. Asylum lawyers and clinicians at low-cost health care centers have similarly heavy caseloads, slim resources, and must work under demanding deadlines that prevent them from obtaining full-scale physical and psychological assessments of their clients.[7] Yet competent and careful documentation may be a lifeline for a client seeking to avoid being returned to the place they were persecuted.

The purpose of this article is to explain how lawyers and doctors work together in the asylum process. The article, first, reviews the demographic composition of asylum seekers; second, describes the standards and procedure used in asylum cases in various industrialized countries; third, describes the use of medical and psychological testimony in asylum cases; and, fourth, suggests ways that medical and legal professionals can work together to improve professional services for asylum applicants.[8]

THE FACE OF ASYLUM

There are over 14 million refugees and asylum seekers in the world today.[9] Asylum seekers alone number more than 1.3 million.[10] In the US, applications for asylum have increased at a staggering rate, from 16,622 in 1985 to a high of 154,464 in 1995,[11] reflecting the mass exodus of boat people from Cuba and Haiti. After the mid-decade surge, asylum applications in the US fell to 41,860 in 1999 due, in part, to the effects of a 1996 law that denied asylum seekers the right to obtain work authorization immediately upon arrival.[12] The backlog of asylum cases in the US in

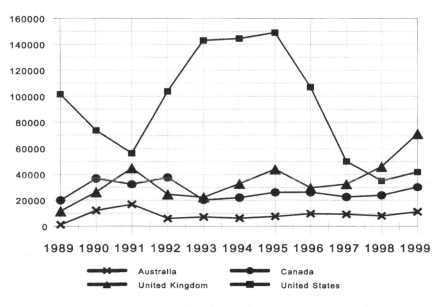

Figure 3.1

July 2000 was 330,290.[13] In Canada, numbers of asylum applications remained relatively constant throughout the 1990s, while the UK experienced a large increase in applications in 1998–99[14] (Figure 3.1). The Australian Department of Immigration and Multicultural Affairs has a quota of about 12,000 immigration permits for refugees applying from overseas, persons found to be suffering gross violations of human rights, displacement or hardship, and in-country asylum seekers.[15] Asylum seekers come from every continent. The ethnicity of asylum seekers varies as country conditions change around the globe.[16] Lawyers representing asylum applicants in the US estimate that at least 50% of their clients are torture victims, and the percentage is closer to 75% if the question has to do with torture of family members.[17] While it is estimated that between 5% and 10% of all foreign-born patients seen in large urban medical centers have experienced some form of torture in their countries of origin,[18] some immigrant groups have been severely affected by torture. The investigators in a five-year study that began in 1998 in Minnesota, for instance, note that only 5% of the hundreds of Somalis they have interviewed have suffered 'no trauma.' The study's preliminary results indicate a prevalence of torture in Somalis (33%) that is at the upper range reported in the professional literature (35%).[19]

Torture is carried out systematically in more than 40 UN member states and is a serious problem in many more.[20] Amnesty International estimates that at least 150 countries practice torture.[21] Governments torture individuals because they belong to the political party that is not in power; participate in public demonstrations; belong to an ethnic group or tribe that is not in power; are suspected of having a different or opposing view from the government or ruling authority; or are related to a person who is politically active.[22] Many people who are subjected to torture are leaders in their countries of origin and this is the very reason they were selected out for persecution. The population of torture survivors is therefore disproportionately well educated and politically aware.[23] Despite their resourcefulness in fleeing to another country, many refugees and asylum applicants continue to suffer ongoing trauma because of separation from families and loved ones, survivor guilt, continuing violence and upheaval in their home countries, and difficulty adapting to their new place of residency due to language impediments, lack of social support networks, poor living conditions and discrimination.

THE ASYLUM PROCESS

While the demand for asylum is high, the approval rate for cases is quite low. In 1999, the US government granted asylum in 13,510 cases (25%), while in 40,463 cases the asylum application was rejected under the one-year filing deadline, referred to the immigration judge or otherwise closed. From January through July 2000, the US government granted asylum in 13,525 cases (27%) and denied, referred or otherwise closed 35,839 cases.[24] Other Western countries had similarly low rates for granting asylum: Australia granted asylum in 24% of adjudicated cases in 1998 and 23% in 1999; France granted asylum in 17.5% of adjudicated cases in 1998 and 19.3% in 1999; Germany granted asylum in 10% of adjudicated cases in 1998 and 13.5% in 1999. The UK had the highest approval rate in adjudicated asylum cases during this time period: 34.6% in 1998 and 72.5% in 1999.[25]

Governments are increasingly resorting to the administrative detention of asylum seekers for individuals who are considered a risk because of use of falsified documentation, previous history of failing to comply with immigration control, or likelihood that they will fail to meet the asylum standard.[26] Asylum seekers who are in jail awaiting the government's determination of their claim have serious barriers to finding effective legal representation or medical attention. The US detains about 16,000 asylum seekers, more than half in local jails, with no provision for medical or psychological treatment and severely curtailed access to legal representation. At any one time, approximately 200 to 500 immigration detainees are unaccompanied minors in the custody of the US Immigration and Naturalization Service (INS).[27] Detainees report difficulty receiving even the most basic medical services, and usually are not given the time or facilities necessary even to get a medical evaluation at their own initiative.[28]

To be granted asylum, a person must meet a statutory definition of a refugee, which in most countries is modeled after the 1951 UN Convention Relating to the Status of

Refugees, as completed by the 1967 Protocol:

> For the purposes of the present convention, the term 'refugee' shall apply to any person who ... owing to well-founded fear of being persecuted for reasons of race, religion, nationality, membership of a particular social group or political opinion, is outside the country of his nationality and is unable, or owing to such fear, is unwilling to avail himself of the protection of that country; or who, not having a nationality and being outside the country of his former habitual residence as a result of such events, is unable or, owing to such fear, is unwilling to return to it.[29]

Countries may choose to emphasize one or more of the Convention grounds for determining refugee status. Under US law, persecution on account of race, religion, nationality, membership in a particular social group, or political opinion are weighted equally and applicants for asylum must show that they have a well-founded fear of persecution based on at least one of these grounds.[30] The Federal Republic of Germany's statutory definition of a person eligible for asylum, on the other hand, includes only persons persecuted for political reasons.[31]

Asylum applications are considered on a case-by-case basis. An individual may apply for asylum affirmatively or may use an asylum claim as a defense to the government's efforts to remove him or her from the country. Typically, the asylum process begins with a hearing by a government caseworker; clients are given an opportunity to appeal a negative ruling to a higher authority or judge.[32]

Persecution under US law is broadly defined as 'a showing that harm or suffering will be inflicted upon [the applicant] in order to punish her for possessing a belief or characteristic the persecutor seeks to overcome,'[33] or as 'the infliction of suffering or harm upon those who differ ... in a way that is regarded as offensive.'[34] Guidelines in the UK note, '[t]here is no universally accepted definition of "persecution" for the purposes of the Convention. The ordinary meaning of the term "persecution" must be taken in its context.'[35]

What constitutes persecution is determined by the finder of fact in each case. Unjustifiable killing, maiming, and physical or psychological torture undoubtedly amount to persecution under the 1951 Convention when perpetrated by an agent of government. Although gender is not included as one of the protected grounds under the 1951 Convention, rape has been equated with torture under certain circumstances.[36] For purposes of asylum, economic deprivation alone does not amount to persecution unless it is individualized and severe or coupled with other evidence of persecution.[37]

Well-founded fear of persecution

Proof of a 'well-founded fear' of persecution is the heart of the asylum case. What constitutes a well-founded fear differs slightly from country to country, but always involves some balance of subjective and objective observation. In the UK, an applicant must show that her well-founded fear is objective.[38] The objective test is met if, measured objectively, there is a 'reasonable likelihood of the fear of persecution being realized then the applicant should return to his country.'[39] Under the US law, an asylum applicant should subjectively demonstrate genuine fear.[40] The fear must be objectively well founded, that is, it must be based on specific facts which would lead to a conclusion that a reasonable person in the applicant's circumstances would fear persecution.[41]

In the US, an applicant may be granted asylum for past persecution, well-founded fear of future persecution, or both. All asylum applicants must show they have a well-founded fear of future persecution. If they can prove past persecution, they are legally presumed to have a well-founded fear.[42] It then falls to the government to prove that, because conditions have changed, the fear arising from past persecution is no longer reasonable or well founded. If the persecution suffered by the applicant was exceptionally severe, asylum may be granted as a humanitarian gesture even if, because of changed circumstances, there is no objective basis for continued fear.[43]

In theory, the applicant's testimony alone is sufficient to establish both the subjective and objective elements of well-founded fear when the testimony is detailed, consistent and believable.[44] In practice, most judges in the US look for evidence of past torture or severe physical injury before granting asylum based on past persecution,[45] and the US Board of Immigration Appeals (BIA) is increasingly emphasizing the importance of documentary and physical evidence, such as documentation of medical treatment.[46]

Credibility: the applicant

The applicant's credibility is the key to establish a well-founded fear of persecution.[47] The practical assumption made by many adjudicators in asylum cases is that the application is fraudulent, and the burden is therefore on the client to establish every fact of the case.[48] The atmosphere surrounding the decision-making process for asylum claims in the UK, for instance, has been described as a 'culture of disbelief.'[49] An asylum applicant's credibility is always at issue in any decision on the merits of an asylum case since cases are decided primarily on the basis of the applicant's own written and oral testimony. Asylum applicants support their cases by providing documentary and physical evidence, such as written death threats, news articles about the facts they are describing, affidavits or correspondence from witnesses within the country of origin, and photographs. Inconsistencies in an applicant's testimony and documentary evidence can lead to a finding that the applicant is not credible.[50]

THE USE OF MEDICAL AND PSYCHOLOGICAL TESTIMONY IN ASYLUM CASES

Medical and psychological evidence verifying the torture victim's injuries or sequelae offers critical support to the asylum case. This evidence serves to educate immigration judges and officials about the effects of torture on the applicant's demeanor and memory of events,[51] and supports the client's credibility when medical and psychological symptoms correspond to their accounts of trauma.[52] The participation of health care workers in the client's asylum case also has therapeutic value because it validates that the client is truthful and believable and has suffered tremendously.[53] Health care professionals working with torture victims assert that documentation of the human rights violations suffered by their patients is as important as treating the resulting symptoms 'because efforts to assess the veracity of an individual's claim are essential to ensuring the person a safe haven ...'[54]

Medical and psychological experts usually offer their expert testimony in writing. Medical reports need to be written in lay language so that they are understandable to the non-medical reader.[55] An ability to clearly communicate how the medical expert used his or her professional skills, training, or expertise to come to the particular conclusions noted in the medical report will also enhance their credibility.[56]

The lawyer in the case may choose to submit the medical/psychological file itself, or may work with the health care professionals to develop an affidavit or a letter in support of the client's application for asylum. Any written submission by physicians or psychologists should contain:

(1) the professional background or experience of the expert

(2) the circumstances under which the client came to be treated

(3) the definition of torture under which the expert is evaluating the client[57]

(4) medical or psychological assessment results including, for instance, a diagnosis of post-traumatic stress disorder under the Diagnostic and Statistical Manual, 4th edn., of the American Psychiatric Association (DSM-IV)[58]

(5) observations of physical/medical symptoms consistent with the client's story[59]

(6) explanation of any potentially inconsistent or detrimental evidence[60]

(7) considerations for the client during the interview or hearing

(8) ongoing treatment and recommendations, and

(9) the signature of the evaluating expert.[61]

The report must explain how these elements support the client's application as a whole – the medical expert's analysis of the information often provides the critical linkages for the government caseworker who is evaluating the legitimacy of the asylum claim.[62]

In the US, while only the client is allowed to participate in the interview with the asylum officer, physicians and psychologists are occasionally requested to testify at the client's asylum hearing if the case is referred to the immigration judge. The professional may testify in person or by telephone, but often only an affidavit is accepted due to the constraints in hearing schedules.[63] Removal hearings are conducted in an adversarial fashion; the role of the government immigration lawyers is to show, usually through cross-examination, that the client has not carried his or her burden of proving that they deserve asylum.[64] The content of the medical professional's oral testimony will be substantially the same as that contained in the written report. The medical professional, however, will be subject to cross-examination by the government immigration lawyers, and may also be questioned by the judge.

On direct examination, questions by the client's lawyer will establish the physician or psychologist's qualifications as an expert witness, the physician or psychologist's experience with the client population, the referral process in the expert's practice, the nature and purpose of standard medical or psychological evaluation, the length and frequency of the client's treatment, observations about the client over the course of treatment, the logical elimination of alternative explanations for client's symptoms, the expert's assessment of the client's condition and how that condition might affect the client's testimony at the hearing.[65] Typical challenges to the physician's or psychologist's expert testimony include lack of sufficient experience, lack of relevant experience, refusal to consider other plausible explanations for client's physical or medical symptoms, and lack of objectivity because of employment as a human rights advocate or examination at the behest of a human rights advocate.[66]

Besides the written report, the examining physician may offer documentary evidence at the hearing, such as X-rays or photographs of the client's injuries. This type of evidence may also prevent the client from having to show the judge or asylum officer their body parts during the hearing.[67] The physician must substantiate the documentary evidence by explaining when and where it was created and verifying its accuracy. Where there are no physical signs of torture – torturers are becoming sophisticated in the use of methods that leave few if any visible marks – the medical expert can provide an independent assessment of the applicant's credibility.[68]

In the UK, the Medical Foundation for the Care of Victims of Torture (Medical Foundation) provides guidelines for doctors who are writing medical reports for asylum applicants who allege that they were tortured.[69] Government caseworkers may request a copy of any medical reports, and the client is advised that the government may draw negative conclusions about an applicant's credibility when a medical report is known to have been prepared but not submitted. Medical reports by themselves are not proof that the applicant has been tortured ('… caseworkers should [not] accept all Medical Foundation reports as prima facie evidence that the applicant has been tortured').[70]

At present, the US INS does not use its own medical experts to contradict the examining physician's testimony.[71] There is a growing trend, however, for the INS to characterize physicians and psychologists from organizations specializing in treatment of torture victims as 'advocates' rather than medical experts[72] and, as such, to discount their testimony.[73] In these situations, physicians and psychologists from organizations that work with torture victims may choose to offer oral testimony at asylum hearings to offer additional weight to their written reports.[74] In some cases, immigration judges are requesting testimony from additional medical experts, including specialists, to establish adequate proof of the client's claims of torture.[75]

PROFESSIONAL COOPERATION IN SUPPORT OF THE ASYLUM APPLICANT

Lawyers and treating physicians or psychologists have different approaches to their work with asylum applicants. The role of the lawyer is to obtain a specific legal status for the client within a set time period, a time period which is often very short.[76] The health care professional, in contrast, is concerned with the medical and psychological healing of the client, a process which may take a very long period of time. Lawyers need to obtain factual information from clients which will support their asylum claim. Health care professionals are less concerned about the specific dates or details of the ill-treatment than they are with the physical or psychological sequelae of such ill-treatment.

Because of these differences in professional function, it is critical for lawyers and medical professionals to communicate with each other about the needs of the client and to educate each other about the purposes of their professional roles. It is also important for the professionals to educate the client regarding their relative roles in the case. Keeping the client informed about the professionals' responsibilities and decisions at all stages in the asylum process is the basis of ethical professional representation; it can also result in the most effective representation. Torture victims, for instance, may not want to retell their story to a lawyer when they have already had to discuss it in depth with their psychologist or physician. The client's frustration may be somewhat alleviated if they understand that the lawyer and the doctor are seeking different kinds of information for different purposes. The client must review the written submissions in their asylum case, including the draft medical report and the asylum application, in order to clarify any misstatements or confusion in the documents before they are submitted to the government.

Legal and medical professionals working with torture victims in asylum cases must obtain a written release from the client in order to share information about their client's case. The release allows the professionals to consult with each other about all aspects of the client's case and the client's well-being. By accessing the medical files, for instance, the lawyer can learn a great deal of background information and thus may be able to conduct interviews that are less repetitive and therefore less difficult for the client. Releases allow medical professionals to provide information helpful to the client's asylum case directly to the lawyer in situations where the client is uncomfortable discussing the facts outside a therapy setting. Before the hearing, the doctor and the lawyer should discuss discrepancies in the client's case and other issues of concern including conditions that may impair the client's ability to testify.

Besides providing evidence in asylum cases, health care professionals, particularly psychologists, can serve as personal support for torture victims. First and foremost, physicians and psychologists provide help and healing for torture victims, many of whom are unable to remember, unable to talk about, or severely retraumatized by describing what they suffered. If applicants are unable to describe their persecution in precise and credible detail to the asylum adjudicator they will lose their case.

Health care workers can help the lawyer prepare the client for the asylum hearing by participating in exercises such as mock hearings with simulated questioning by a person posing as an immigration officer or judge.[77] In such an exercise, the health care professional has an opportunity to observe the client's demeanor in order to provide needed emotional support as well as to help the lawyer and judge better understand the client's state of mind. At the actual hearing, lawyers who represent torture victims can ask to call the physician or psychologist to testify *before* the client takes the stand, so that the doctor can stay in the hearing room as a physical presence in support of the client during his or her own testimony.[78]

Communication between professionals is the key to successfully representing torture victims in their asylum cases. Advance preparation by the lawyer and medical professionals can go a long way toward providing the evidence necessary to support the client's asylum application, as well as addressing the fears of the client faced with this intimidating process.

CONCLUSION

Medical and legal professionals play a critical role in defending the rights of asylum seekers, especially torture victims. By working together to represent the best interests of the client, these professionals can secure a safe haven for their clients – the first step in putting their lives back together.

ACKNOWLEDGEMENT

The author gratefully acknowledges the contribution of Martha H Rickey to this chapter.

REFERENCES

1   Kathleen Antolak. Recognizing and caring for survivors of torture, unpublished training materials, 2000, available from the author
2   Physicians for Human Rights, Medical Testimony on Victims of Torture: A Physician's Guide to Political Asylum Cases 13, Boston, 1991

3 Piwowarczyk L, Moreno A, Grodin M. Health care of torture survivors, 284 JAMA No. 5 (2 August 2000) at p 541; Interview with Michele Garnett McKenzie and Jennifer Prestholdt, Immigration Attorneys, Minnesota Advocates for Human Rights, in Minneapolis, Minn. (4 May 2000) (hereinafter, 'McKenzie and Prestholdt interview')

4 Interview with Michele Garnett McKenzie, Immigration Attorney, Minnesota Advocates for Human Rights, in Minneapolis, Minn. (15 November 2000)

5 Physicians for Human Rights, *supra* note 2

6 Deborah E Anker. Law of Asylum in the United States, 104, Paul T Lufkin (managing ed.), 3rd edn. 1999

7 McKenzie and Prestholdt interview, *supra* note 3

8 For guidance on the medical or psychological treatment of torture survivors, cf., e.g., Vince Iacopino, Ozkalipici O, Scholar C *et al*, Manual on the effective investigation and documentation of torture and other cruel, inhuman and degrading treatment (The Istanbul Protocol), http://www.phrusa.org (accessed 24 October 2000); Culpepper L, Primary care treatment guide for post-traumatic stress disorder: Treatment of post-traumatic stress disorder expert consensus guideline series. J Clin Psych 1999; 60

9 US Committee for Refugees, World Refugee Survey 2000. The terms 'refugee' and 'asylum seeker' both refer to individuals who are seeking protection from returning to countries where they will face persecution. The difference between refugees and asylees is based on the countries where they apply for protection and are processed. Refugees are processed from without national boundaries, and asylum seekers apply and are processed within the country. This article therefore addresses the issues faced by asylum seekers who are still trying to prove their case, not those of refugees who already have legal status upon arrival

10 United Nations High Commissioner for Refugees, www.unhcr.ch/statist/99oview/tab101.pdf (accessed 25 August 2000)

11 Refugee Reports, Vol. 21, No. 2, 2000, available at: http://www.refugees.org/world/articles/asylum_rr00_2.htm (accessed 2 October 2000)

12 Matthew Wilch. Detect, detain, deter, deport. Refugees, Vol. 2, No. 119, 2000, at p 18 (UNHCR, Geneva 2000) (citing the Illegal Immigration Reform and Immigrant Responsibility Act of 1996 (IIRIRA), Pub. L. No. 104-208, 110 Stat. 3009 (1996)). For more information on IIRIRA, see: Kristen B Rosati, The United Nations Convention Against Torture: A Detailed Examination of the Convention as an Alternative for Asylum Seekers, 97-12 Immigration Briefings 1, 1997

13 United States Immigration and Naturalization service, 'Asylum', July 2000, available at: http://www.ins.gov/graphics/aboutins/statistics/msrjuly00/ASYLUM.HTM (accessed 2 Oct 2000)

14 UK Home Office, Asylum Statistics, June 2000, available at: http://www.homeoffice.gov.uk/rds/areas/immif.htm

15 Australian Department of Immigration and Multicultural Affairs, DIMA Fact Sheet 2, Key Facts in Immigration (2000), available at: http://www.immi.gov.au/facts/02key-2.htm (accessed 28 June 2000)

16 In 1999, for instance, the top four countries of origin for asylum applicants in the United States were China (10%), Somalia (8%), Haiti (6%), and Indonesia (6%), while in Canada they were Sri Lanka (10%), China (8%), Pakistan (8%), and Hungary (5%). Ray Wilkinson, Give me … your huddled masses … , Refugees, Vol 2. No 119, at pp 4, 7 (UNHCR, Geneva 2000). The Federal Republic of Yugoslavia continued to be the main country of origin of asylum seekers in Europe in year 2000, accounting for 11.7% of all new applications submitted, followed by Iraq (9.0%), the Islamic Republic of Iran (7.2%), Afghanistan (6.8%), Turkey (5.3%), the Russian Federation (4.4%), China (3.2%), Somalia (2.9%), and Sri Lanka (2.8%). Registration and Statistics Unit, United Nations High Commissioner for Refugees, 'Asylum Applications in Europe, January–July 2000,' Geneva 2000, available at http://www.unhcr.ch/statst/00h1asyl/jul00asy.pdf

17 McKenzie and Prestholdt interview, *supra* note 3; Telephone interview with Mary McCarthy, Director, Midwest Immigrant and Human Rights Center, from Chicago, Ill. (15 September 2000) (hereinafter 'McCarthy interview')

18 Alejandro Moreno, Michael Grodin, The not-so-silent marks of torture, 284 JAMA at p 538 (2 August 2000)

19 Electronic communication from James Jaranson, Investigator for the Refugee and Populations Study of Somalis and Ethiopians (Oromos) in the Twin Cities, Division of Epidemiology at the U of M School of Public Health, funded by the National Institute of Mental Health, from Minneapolis (21 September 2000)

20 International Rehabilitation Council for Torture victims (IRCT), Torture is a Global Problem, available at: http://www.irct.org (accessed 25 September 2000)

21 Amnesty International, Campaign to Stop Torture, www.stoptorture.org (accessed 24 October 2000)

22 Antolak, *supra* note 1

23 Ibid.

24 United States Immigration and Naturalization service, 'Asylum', July 2000, available at: http://www.ins.gov/graphics/aboutins/statistics/msrjuly00/ASYLUM.HTM (accessed 2 October 2000). 'Cases' may involve more than one person

25 In Australia, the government rejected 7980 out of 10,470 adjudicated asylum cases in 1998, and 6610 out of 8550. The French Government rejected 18,770 out of 22,750 in 1998 and 19,490 out of 24,150 in 1999. The German Government rejected 130,080 out of 143,940 in 1998 and 83,730 out of 96,770 in 1999. The UK rejected 17,470 out of 26,730 in 1998 and 7730 out of 28,150 in 1999. Most of the increase in approvals of asylum in the UK in 1999 was the result of individuals fleeing the conflict in Kosovo. UN High Commissioner for

Refugees, Refugees and Others of Concern to UNHCR – 1999 Statistical Overview, Tables V.8 and V.10, 2000, available at: http://www.unhcr.ch/statist/99oview/tab508.pdf (accessed 3 October 2000)

26 See, e.g., UN Commission on Human Rights, 'Report of the Working Group on Arbitrary Detention, Report on the visit of the Working Group to the UK on the issue of immigrants and asylum seekers,' E/CN.4/1999/63/Add.3 (1999); Medical Foundation for the Care of Victims of Torture, 'Comments on Detention: New Forms and Procedures' October 1999, available at: http://www.torturecare.org.uk/pubbrf10.htm#UK (accessed 4 January 2001)

27 UN Commission on Human Rights 'Written statement submitted by Human Rights Watch', January 1999

28 McKenzie and Prestholdt interview, *supra* note 3

29 Article 1(A)(2), UN Convention relating to the Status of Refugees, 189 UNTS 150, entered into force 22 April 1954

30 INA Section 101(a)(42)(A), 8 USC Section 1101(a)(42)(A)

31 Article 16AI of the Basic Law, as amended in June 1993

32 For a discussion of comparative asylum procedure and practice see: Helene Lambert, Seeking Asylum: Comparative Law and Practice in Selected European Countries (Int'l Studies in Human Rights, Vol. 37, The Netherlands, 1995)

33 See Guevara-Flores v. INS, 786 F.2nd 1242 (5th Cir. 1986)

34 See Desir v. Ilchert, 840 F.2nd 723, 727 (9th Cir. 1988); Matter of Acosta, 19 I&N Dec. 211,222 (BIA 1985)

35 UK Home Office, Immigration and Nationality Directorate, Law and Policy. Chapter 1, Section 2, Part 8, 'Persecution' available at: http://www.ind.homeoffice.gov.uk/default.asp?PageId = 927#annexa (accessed 4 January 2001)

36 Generally, where the rape was government sanctioned or sponsored. See: Nancy Kelly, Commentary: Political rape as persecution: a legal perspective. 52 J Am Med Women's Assoc 188, Fall 1997

37 Minnesota Advocates for Human Rights. 1999. Fourteenth Annual Asylum Conference 12, held at University of Minn. Law School, Minneapolis, Minn. (21 May 1999)

38 UK Home Office, Immigration and Naturalization Directorate, Law and Policy, available at: http://www.ind.homeoffice.gov.uk/default.asp? PageId = 87 (accessed 4 January 2001)

39 UK Home Office, Immigration and Nationality Directorate, Law and Policy, available at: http://www.ind.homeoffice.gov.uk/default.asp?PageId = 927 ('Caseworkers must assess objectively in each individual case whether there is a reasonable likelihood of the fear of persecution being realised should the applicant be returned to his country of origin. The aim is to identify the genuine refugee as quickly as possible. Applying the test of reasonable likelihood if the considerations are

finely balanced, the benefit of the doubt should always be given to the applicant ...')

40 See INS v. Cardoza-Fonseca, 480 US 421 (1987)

41 See Matter of Mogharrabi, 19 I&N Dec. 439 (BIA 1987)

42 8 CFR Section 208, 13(b)(1)(i)

43 Davis, Wendy B, Angela D. Atchue, *supra* note 35 at p 84

44 Deborah E Anker. Law of Asylum in the United States, *supra* note 6 at p 91

45 Davis, Wendy B, Angela D Atchue. No Physical Harm, No Asylum: Denying a Safe Haven for Refugees, 5 Tex F C.L. & C.R. 81, 83 2000

46 Deborah E Anker. Law of Asylum in the United States, *supra* note 6 at pp 92, 100 (quoting In Re: S-M-J-, Interim Dec. 3303, at 5–6 (BIA 1997), that '[i]f the applicant does not provide such information [e.g. documentation of medical treatment], an explanation should be given as to why such information was not presented ... The absence of such corroborating evidence can lead to a finding that an applicant has failed to meet her burden of proof.')

47 Kirsten Schlenger. The nuts and bolts of representing an asylum applicant. In: Corporate Law and Practice 1998, at p 242 (PLI Corp. Law and Practice Course, Handbook Series No. 108, PLI Order No. B0-0055, October 1998)

48 McKenzie and Prestholdt interview, *supra* note 3

49 Peter W Billings, A comparative analysis of administrative and adjudicative systems for determining asylum claims. 52 Admin L Rev pp 253, 277 (Winter 2000)

50 Caseworkers in the UK are instructed to give the applicant an opportunity to explain the inconsistencies. 'Where the applicant has been given no opportunity to explain inconsistencies, care should be taken about using the inconsistencies to question credibility.' UK Home Office, Immigration and Nationality Directorate, Law and Policy. Chapter 1, Section 2, Part 11 'Assessing the Claim: Credibility', available at:
http://www.ind.homeoffice.gov.uk/default.asp?PageId = 927#annexa (accessed 4 January 2001)

51 Physicians for Human Rights, *supra* note 2 at p 1

52 Douglas A Shenson. A primary care clinic for the documentation and treatment of human rights abuses, 11 JGIM p 535 (1996)

53 Center for victims of torture. Written testimony for asylum, unpublished training materials, 1999, available from the author

54 Shenson, *supra* note 52 at p 533; Interview with Dr Rosa Garcia-Peltoniemi, Clinical Director for the Center for Victims of Torture, St. Paul, Minn. (22 May 2000)

55 Stanley L Brodsky. Testifying in Court: Guidelines and Maxims for the Expert Witness, 47 (Washington, DC, 1991)

56 Ibid. at pp 98–99

57 The most comprehensive definition of torture is contained in Article I of the Convention against Torture, which states that: 'the term "torture" means any act

by which severe pain or suffering, whether physical or mental, is intentionally inflicted on a person for such purposes as obtaining from him or a third person information or a confession, punishing him for an act he or a third person has committed or is suspected of having committed, or intimidating or coercing him or a third person, or for any reason based on discrimination of any kind, when such pain or suffering is inflicted by or at the instigation of or with the consent or acquiescence of a public official or other person acting in an official capacity. It does not include pain or suffering arising only from, inherent in or incidental to lawful sanctions.' Convention against Torture and Other Cruel, Inhuman or Degrading Treatment or Punishment, GA res. 39/46 [Annex 39 UN GAOR Supp. (No. 51) at p 197, UN Doc. A/39/51 (1984)], entered into force June 26, 1987

58 American Psychiatric Ass'n, Diagnostic and Statistical Manual of Mental Disorders (DSM-IV), 4th edn. 1994

59 In the US, for instance, the asylum client must provide evidence of his claim when available or explain its lack of availability. In Re: S-M-J-, Interim Dec. 3303, at pp 5–6 (BIA 1997)

60 The immigration judge in the US draws adverse inferences from the applicant's failure to refute or explain the negative conclusions that can be drawn from medical or forensic reports. In Re: O-D-, Interim Decision 3334 (BIA, 1998)

61 Andrea Northwood, Content of Asylum Letter, Center for Victims of Torture, unpublished training materials, 1999, available from the author

62 Shenson, *supra* note 52 at p 533

63 McCarthy interview, *supra* note 17; interview with Dr Rosa Garcia Peltoniemi, Clinical Director, Center for Victims of Torture, St. Paul, Minn. (22 May 2000) ('The CVT is now encouraging personal testimony in every case.') (hereinafter 'Garcia interview')

64 The government lawyer will try to discredit the medical expert's report regardless of whether the expert testifies in person. Careful preparation of written testimony will help prevent the government's ability to undermine the expert's testimony

65 Andrea Northwood, Direct Examination, Center for Victims of Torture, unpublished training materials, 1999, available from the author

66 See, e.g., Stanley L. Brodsky, *supra* note 55; Garcia interview, *supra* note 63

67 Interview with Dr Kathy Antolak, Staff Physician, Center for Victims of Torture, Minneapolis, Minn. (5 June 2000)

68 Physicians for Human Rights, *supra* note 2 at p 13

69 See Medical Foundation for the Care of Victims of Torture, Comments of the Medical Foundation on the White Paper entitled Fairer, Faster and Firmer, A Modern Approach to Immigration and Asylum, October 1998, available at: http://www.torturecare.org.uk/pubbrf10.htm#UK (accessed 4 January 2001)

70 Medical reports can be submitted with the initial application or separately on appeal. See UK Home Office, Immigration and Nationality Directorate, Law

and Policy, Chapter 17, Section 3 'The Medical Foundation' available at: http://www.homeoffice.gov.uk

71 McKenzie and Prestholdt interview, *supra* note 3

72 McKenzie and Prestholdt interview, *supra* note 3; Garcia interview, *supra* note 63

73 Garcia interview, *supra* note 63

74 Ibid.

75 Interview with Paula Schwartzbauer, attorney, Centro Legal, Minneapolis, Minn. (15 September 2000) (immigration judge requested lawyer to obtain the additional expert opinion of a urology specialist regarding her client's claim of genital torture, despite evidence previously submitted through the testimony of the Center for Victims of Torture)

76 The Illegal Immigration Reform and Immigrant Responsibility Act of 1996 ('IIRIRA'), INA Section 208(a)(2)(B) and (D), bars an asylum application not filed within one year of the applicant's last arrival, except under extraordinary circumstances. Under this tight time restriction, if a client delays in seeking professional representation, the lawyer may have an extremely short deadline for filing the case

77 McCarthy interview, *supra* note 17

78 Ibid. Witnesses are prohibited from observing prior testimony in court, to avoid prejudicing the nature of their testimony

4

DOCTORS AND TORTURE

Ann Somerville, Hernan Reyes, Michael Peel

INTRODUCTION

The main focus of this book is on doctors examining alleged victims of torture with a view to documenting their injuries and giving an expert opinion on the consistency between the injuries and the history. However, it must always be stressed that the absence of physical findings must never be construed as evidence of absence of torture. Information and expert opinion from medical examinations can then be used both to assist in the prosecution of perpetrators, and to help the patient seek asylum status in another country. The work involves both awareness of human rights issues and medical ethics. These are not necessarily the same although there is considerable overlap between principles of modern medical ethics and concepts of basic human rights since both focus, in different ways, on ensuring respect for the individual. Furthermore, although awareness of notions of human rights is a historically recent development, it has exercised considerable influence on the evolution of modern ethical standards. In practice, this means that a breach of any international standards of human rights by medical personnel is also very likely to be a contravention of medical ethics.

Human rights are international legal principles that were first fully formulated in the Universal Declaration of Human Rights in 1948, and that go back beyond the philosophy of the French and American Revolutions. They define the actions that States cannot commit, whether or not they are democratically elected, such as imprisonment without due process, torture, and slavery. The obligation to observe human rights falls on all citizens, but particularly those acting in an official capacity.[1] Doctors thus have duties in addition to their traditional role as healers. They also have a duty to protect the dignity of all those with whom they have professional contact, and to do their part in the investigation of human rights abuses brought to their attention. Medical ethics are the moral principles that regulate the interrelationship between doctors and their patients. The idea that doctors owe special duties to the sick and vulnerable has existed in all societies for centuries. In the Western tradition of medicine, it was first formulated in the so-called Hippocratic Oath more than 2500 years ago. Similar principles, emphasising compassion and a duty of care, have traditionally been articulated in other cultures. Doctors should already be aware of the basic principles.[2] How they relate to possible situations of torture is described below.

RELEVANT ETHICAL PRINCIPLES

It is important to emphasise at the outset that medical ethics apply to all professional activities undertaken by physicians. Ethical standards should not differ, therefore, when doctors are seeing private patients in expensive clinics or employed in prisons, police stations, immigrants' detention centres or refugee camps. This means that doctors' ethical duties may sometimes come into conflict with rules and regulations applied in some of these contexts. Internationally, it is widely accepted, however, that doctors should give priority to observing agreed ethical standards and should not be pressured by contractual or other regulations to compromise either their conscience or their ethical duties.

Respect for autonomy

Doctors must allow their patients to express their autonomy. The fact that a person is a suspected, or even convicted, 'criminal', or 'terrorist' does not change this ethical obligation to respect individuals' fundamental right to decide what is done to their bodies. Unpressured consent is difficult to ensure in any situation where the patient is already very restricted in expressing choices. Nevertheless, even in a prison setting, a patient still generally has to give valid consent to medical interventions and to non-medical procedures, such as intimate body searches, which may in certain specific cases be performed by health personnel. Nevertheless, no ethical principle is absolute and inflexible. Clearly, some examinations or treatments may have to be provided in order to prevent foreseeable threats to public health in detention centres but these should not involve greater limitations on the individual than occurs in the rest of society where measures to prevent transmission of infectious diseases can also impinge on patients' self-determination. Thus, in cases where patients in the community would be given a choice about treatment options or elective procedures, the same should apply in prisons. There are daily examples, however, of this principle being breached in prisons. For example, there have been many allegations that in Sri Lanka, Tamil detainees have blood taken from them without consent 'to replace the blood that they have spilled'. In one case, a detainee said that he was told that he would be released if he said to the doctor that he was giving blood freely. He gave the blood but was detained for a further four months before he was released, and the release was unrelated to the blood donation. Doctors and other health care professionals must make sure that there is genuine consent in all circumstances where best practice would require informed consent in a community setting. Properly informed and unpressured consent is even more important when individuals appear to be agreeing to a procedure, such as blood or tissue donation, which is not in their own health interests. The World Medical Association has determined that prisoners should not be used for organ donations (except if the donation is to a member of their immediate family), as they are not in a situation where consent can be given freely, and may be submitted to coercion.

Confidentiality

Confidentiality is not an absolute right for any patient but must always be respected as much in the prison context as it is in the community. If, for legal reasons, clinical information is likely to be divulged, this must be explained to the patient at the outset of the consultation. Legal reasons are not always legitimate reasons, as far as medical ethics are concerned.[3] Doctors as a rule should always insist that examination of detained patients be conducted in privacy and out of earshot of guards or policemen or any other non-medical staff. The presence of a chaperone may be required, however, when gender difference between patient and physician so requires.

Duty of care

Doctors working in places of detention owe a duty of care to the people they examine or treat, regardless of the purpose of that examination or treatment. This means that doctors employed by the authorities to work for the military, the police, the prison service, or in similar roles are likely to encounter problems of dual responsibilities. As well as the duties owed to any patient, they may be expected to play a disciplinary role, becoming involved in maintaining order or monitoring punishments. Punishments that are quite obviously deleterious to prisoners' health should not be permitted.[4] They may have little choice and few powers to protect their patients from abuse. If conscripted, doctors could be working within a regime which they do not support, and which has a severe disciplinary code. As mentioned previously, however, doctors must do their best to ensure that their ethical duties take precedence over any legal or contractual obligations.

Health professionals have an ethical responsibility to offer an equivalent quality of medical care to detainees as is available to the general population. It also is a breach of the human rights of the prisoners if the authorities deny them medical services that are available in the local community.[5] For example, the formularies used by the prison service should be similar to those used in civilian practice. In many countries, this is not the case and prison doctors have a difficult task to ensure that their patients are not routinely assigned sub-optimal treatments. One consequence of this neglect of patients is that victims learn to mistrust doctors, leading them to avoid seeking medical help after imprisonment.[6]

There may be other reasons for prisoners not to trust the prison doctor. Doctors working in prisons are often underpaid, ill-considered by their superiors, and receive no training on prison health issues. As a result they are not very motivated in performing their jobs, which leads the prisoners to mistrust their services. Prison doctors in situations where torture is a reality will also be, rightly or wrongly, as accomplices of 'the system' and also be mistrusted.

Whistleblowing

Doctors must speak out when they become aware of unethical or abusive practices. It is widely recognised, however, that the pressures a doctor might be under to conform to bad practice are immense. Sometimes, wider issues must be considered beyond medical ethics, including the practical consequences such as whether disclosure of abuse will put the victim or the victim's family in great danger. Physicians must also consider their own safety and may need to work with other professionals, such as lawyers to minimise the risks of reprisals. This is a position of considerable vulnerability for which support must come from national medical associations or the international community.[7]

In one of the countries of the former Soviet Union, a prison doctor was confronted with the reality of incoming prisoners having been visibly brutalised or even tortured in pre-custody. As his position was precarious (he was under the direct authority of the military command of the prison) he feared for his own safety and that of his family if he were to 'blow the whistle'. The solution he found was to document each case he received in a separate, privately kept, notebook. He said that the day there was an outside investigation, with guarantees for the safety of those testifying, he could thus come forward and produce his evidence. In the meantime, however, he felt he had no choice but to continue working within the system.

ETHICS AND TORTURE

The United Nations Principles of Medical Ethics states:

> Principle 2
> 'It is a gross contravention of medical ethics, as well as an offence under applicable international instruments, for health personnel, particularly physicians, to engage, actively or passively, in acts which constitute participation in, complicity in, incitement to or attempts to commit torture or other cruel, inhuman or degrading treatment or punishment.'[8]

The World Medical Association uses a broader definition of torture compared to that of the United Nations Convention against Torture.[9] It is 'the deliberate, systematic or wanton infliction or mental suffering ... for any ... reason'. Thus it is unethical if the intention is to cause unnecessary pain – mental or physical – irrespective of why the pain is caused or by whom. However, the definition of torture is evolving in case law, for example in the European Court of Human Rights,[10] and actions that are now considered to be torture might not have been so 20 years ago.

While it is clear that doctors should not collaborate with or facilitate any kind of deliberate abuse, 'participation' in this context does not just mean actively assisting torturers or standing by when a person is being tortured. There are many situations in which a doctor's professional duties may bring him or her in contact with torture, including:

- examining individuals on arrival at an institution of detention,
- providing medical treatment services in places of detention,
- advising on fitness to be punished,
- advising on methods of torture,
- actively helping in carrying out torture,

- medical research using detainees as subjects,

- medical participation in external visits to detention centres,

- official documentation of detainees in case of allegations of torture,

- treatment of those who have recently been released,

- investigation of allegations of torture by those no longer detained,

- documentation of allegations of torture for asylum purposes.

'Involvement', therefore, relates to a range of medical activities, some of which are entirely ethical but many of which have a strong potential to draw doctors into an unethical, collusive relationship with gross abusers of human rights. Even apparently innocuous activities, such as treating those who have been recently released, for example, may draw health professionals into an unethical conspiracy of silence about the prevalence of torture in detention. These and other aspects of medical involvement are explored more fully below.

Examining individuals on arrival at an institution of detention

Prisoners should be examined when they arrive at a place of detention.[11] This is principally to identify pre-existing illnesses of the patient. It should be used to ensure continuation of care, for example the prescription of drugs for diabetes or asthma. If the medication is available in the community, or the patient brings his or her own supplies, it is unethical to deny the treatment. This examination must not be used to identify physical or psychological weaknesses to help any interrogators.

There is also an opportunity to document any injuries on arrival, although such injuries can be easily attributed by the authorities as being for example 'due to scuffles resisting arrest'. Nevertheless, pressure on doctors to falsify reports at this stage is generally less common than in other situations. It is permissible for the authorities to use 'reasonable force' to arrest someone, especially if there is a threat to the arresting officers or bystanders. It is for the courts to decide whether the force used was 'reasonable' and proportionate to the circumstances, but doctors can assist the process by ensuring thorough documentation. When the injuries could not possibly have been caused in the way described by the arresting officers, or are highly unlikely to have been so, the doctor is required to say so.

The initial examination will also provide a baseline in case of there be any subsequent allegations of assault. A succession of injuries documented by doctors on consecutive days can be clear evidence of torture.[10] There is generally an assumption that, once a person is in the custody of the authorities, it is for them to explain any injuries that occur subsequently. Detainees do sometimes riot or try to escape, but the force used to control the situation must be the minimum necessary.[11]

Providing medical treatment services in places of detention

The commonest complaint by victims of torture about doctors was that when they needed medical attention it was summary, and given without care or compassion. However, one patient said:

'The army doctor was very caring. He told the soldiers not to give me any more electric shocks when they interrogated me, and to give me more food as I had lost too much weight.'

Even though apparently displaying compassion for the prisoner, this attitude on the part of the doctor shows an unacceptable tolerance of the perpetuation of abuse.

If medical treatment is required of a person who is due to be interrogated, the ethical principles hold. The medical treatment of whatever nature must come first, including hospitalisation or use of psychotropic medication. Irrespective of the pressure or urgency placed on the doctor by the interviewers, the patient must be treated fully and not just 'patched up'.[6] The interviewing authorities must be told that the person is unfit for interview either for a specified time or until further notice.

For example, in South Africa, under the apartheid regime, a team of doctors refused to allow detainees held under security rules who had been on hunger strike to be returned to the prison.[12] Some physicians argue that it is more humane to accede to police demands, because documentation of the torture might lead to further torture for the detainee.[13] However, this policy may be in the short-term interests of the individual, but will not benefit the individual in the longer term, nor any other detainees who will be tortured.

Hunger strikes are a particularly difficult situation for doctors to deal with. Most fasting prisoners do so for two or three weeks, and those of them rarely suffer any harm.[14] As they go on longer, the risks to the hunger striker increase.[15] In an ideal situation, an independent doctor will have explained the risks of prolonged hunger strike, and taken instructions on what the person wants to happen if he or she ceases to be capable of rational thought.[16] This should happen in an environment where the patient's confidentiality can be respected, and where he or she can be protected from undue pressure from political colleagues. In cases where prison doctors have been following hunger strikers before and during the fast, and know what the patients' positions and convictions are, physicians should respect the principles stated in the Declaration of Malta on hunger strikes.[17] This declaration allows physicians to act in the best perceived interests of their patients, while respecting autonomy. If a physician is called upon to take care of a hunger striker already in a comatose state, he or she will have no choice and will have to provide resuscitation. A physician should not rely on what amounts to 'hearsay' in such cases. The opinions of the immediate family should be taken into consideration, but are not paramount. Neither the opinions of the authorities nor those of the patient's political colleagues should be given any weight.

Advising on fitness to be punished

The Standard Minimum Rules for the Treatment of Prisoners[18] advise that:

'The medical officer is to be consulted before implementing any punishment that may be prejudicial to the physical or mental health of a prisoner.'

More than anything else, this reflects the prevailing attitudes in 1957 when this was written, and that there was little medical involvement in the drafting. The requirement does not exist in the 1988 Body of Principles.[11]

For a doctor to say that a person is fit for punishment is to condone starving a patient, assaulting or mutilating the patient, or, at worst, killing him or her. For a profession that is dedicated to the relief of pain and suffering, this is unethical, regardless of any crime that the person has committed. A doctor's involvement in any punishment that could jeopardise the health of a patient is ethically unacceptable. The medical profession must press to eliminate their role in punishment. Even though a doctor has not been involved in the ordering of punishment, he or she can still intervene when the health of a prisoner is being damaged by the punishment.

Solitary confinement is a particularly complex issue. It can be instituted for many reasons, including punishment. However, it can be distressing for the individual, and separate him or her from colleagues who can witness the consequences of ill-treatment and might be able to ask for help. The European Committee for the Prevention of Torture has described prolonged solitary confinement as inhuman and degrading.[19]

Advising on methods of torture

In some countries, doctors are advising government agencies about methods of torture. They are advising on ways of suspending people so that the risk of nerve damage in the arms is minimised. They are developing drugs that cause pain and sickness with no therapeutic potential.[20] It does not need to be stressed how unethical such actions are. Sometimes doctors might be merely short-sighted about the potential misuse of their discoveries or they may deliberately wish to distance themselves from the end-usage of their research. Research that appears to be straightforward, such as into the effects of trauma, can still be of benefit to torturers and doctors involved in research have an ethical obligation to be aware about the potential misuse of their work.

Actively helping in carrying out torture

There were many reports from South America in the 1980s of around 50% of survivors of torture telling of doctors standing in the torture room saying 'yes, he can take a bit more', 'why not try this?', and giving injections, presumably to lower the victim's resistance.[21] There are still such reports coming in, particularly from the Middle East,[22] but the direct involvement of doctors in torture in this way seems to be much less. Presumably as torture is being used as a means of intimidating populations (ethnic cleansing, mass rapes, burning people in their houses, etc.), and there is less of a pretence of gaining information,[20] the use of a valuable resource such as a doctor becomes unnecessary. This is not the place to debate whether there can be any justification for torture. The issue has been widely debated elsewhere.[7] Torture is morally and legally wrong, and it is not an effective way of gaining reliable information from someone who holds vital secrets. Doctors who participate in torture should be prosecuted in the local courts, and where this is not possible, they should be brought to court anywhere in the world when they leave their country, as with all torturers. The medical profession as a whole has a duty to encourage the prosecution of colleagues who are involved in torture.

Participating in torture is not just standing in the room while a person is being beaten. The psychiatrists under the Soviet system who 'diagnosed' illness in dissidents and treated it with powerful psychotropic drugs were equally guilty in participating in torture.[23] There are reports that abuse of psychiatric treatment is still happening in China.[24]

Medical research using detainees as subjects

Detainees have been abused as subjects of medical research in many places, the most infamous being the concentration camps in Nazi Germany and the 'medicalised' military research done on prisoners by the Japanese. From a researcher's point of view, detainees are an easy population to investigate. However, it would be very difficult to ensure that consent to participate is freely given in such an environment. There may be health benefits to individuals who are genuinely willing to help medical research. In principle, detainees should only be involved in research which is aimed at improving the physical or mental health of people in that category. For example, in the past, some useful research was carried out on the health effects of the prison diet with the aim of improving the overall health of detainees. All research must be independently authorised by a properly formulated ethics committee.[7]

Medical visits to detention centres

Part of the protection mechanism for detainees is the opportunity for independent experts, including doctors, to visit people in detention and, if necessary, examine them. In contrast with the previous examples of involvement, this is a very positive way that doctors can contribute to the elimination of torture. Nevertheless, it is important that such visits be carried out by trained personnel and according to pre-agreed protocols. Also that care must be taken to obtain detainees' agreement if information gained from such visits is likely to be published or otherwise made public.[25]

Organisations such as the International Committee of the Red Cross (ICRC) and the European Committee for the Prevention of Torture (CPT) have been visiting detention centres for many years. Both have strict rules of confidentiality in order to gain access to detainees, so there has been little published about their methodologies. Medical members of other NGOs may also have the opportunity to visit detainees, and it is essential that they do not jeopardise their own safety, that of their team members, or that of the detainees.

Official documentation of detainees in case of allegations of torture

Another complaint about doctors from survivors of torture was that they refused to listen to allegation of torture, saying that their responsibility was only to treat. In many countries there is pressure on doctors to deny that torture has occurred by providing negative medical reports,[13] or documenting wounds without expressing an opinion on cause. When such acts happen at official instigation, it helps to sustain the culture of impunity in which torture thrives. It makes it much harder for survivors to take cases against torturers, and it gives the authorities ammunition to use against human rights organisations which are trying to assemble accurate portfolios about incidents of torture.

The ethics of medical report writing are clear. Irrespective of the role of the person requesting the report, it must be accurate, thorough, and impartial. Statements such as 'I did not find any evidence of torture' following an inadequate examination, are disingenuous and ethically unacceptable. One of the reasons for developing the Istanbul Protocol[4] was to provide a consensus of what was necessary to provide an expert opinion on whether the patient had been tortured or not. Anything omission from the Protocol must be noted and explained. When there are two disagreeing reports, one of which has followed the Protocol and the other did not, it is the former that must be given more weight legally. It must always be stressed that the absence of physical signs cannot necessarily be taken as evidence that torture has not taken place.

Treatment of those who have recently been released

When brought someone who has recently been released from detention and is injured, whether through torture or not, a doctor has the choice of behaving actively or passively, ethically or unethically, and he or she can do this intentionally or unintentionally,[22] although it is not always easy for doctors to know what the more ethical alternative should be.

The doctor can simply turn the patient away. In many countries, victims of torture are turned away from medical care once it is known that their ill-health or injuries are a consequence of being detained. In some cases this could be in the best interests of the patient, because the doctor knows that security personnel are active in the hospital, and complaining to the doctor of ill-treatment in detention might put the patient at risk of further detention. It is also possible that the doctor believes that this will avoid him or her taking any responsibility for the welfare of the individual. There were cases in South Africa and Chile[26] of clinics being raided by the police or the army, looking for files of patients who have been treated for injuries following demonstrations that were broken up by them. These doctors put themselves at risk by protecting confidentiality, and others might turn patients away rather than be so brave. However, the Declaration of Tokyo[27] states that the doctor must not condone or tolerate the torture, but doctors should also be aware of the impact of their actions for others. In some situations, lateral thinking may be required so that doctors can fulfil their duties to report (possibly to an overseas expert organisation) without placing torture victims at even greater risk.[28]

Investigation of allegations of torture by those no longer detained

There are an increasing number of NGOs around the world documenting local human rights abuses, including allegations of torture by those who have been assaulted at home by the authorities, or recently released from detention. There are a number of guidelines available to help with this[4,28] and organisations which can give advice, such as IRCT. Key points include:

- the safety and security of the survivors of torture and the investigating team must be protected,[25]

- those interviewing survivors of torture, whether lawyers or health care professionals, must have appropriate training and experience,

- there should be access to physical and psychological treatment services for those whose health has been affected, nothing must be written that could allow specific individuals to be identified, without expressing consent,

- reports on individuals must be independent and impartial, and not appear to support either side,

- documentation must be written in calm, neutral language.

Documentation of allegations of torture for asylum purposes

Allegations of torture are often documented for asylum purposes. Torture is documented as evidence to support a claim that the person is entitled to refugee status. It is important to recognise that a person can have been tortured and not be eligible for asylum, and many people who have not been tortured are eligible. The need for ongoing care and treatment can also be used to support a request for leave to remain on compassionate grounds. The legal test required for asylum claims is much lower than that necessary in a criminal case, or even a civil claim.[29] A medical report should still be accurate, thorough, and impartial. There is no justification for padding out a weak case in order to gain asylum for whom the doctor feels sympathetic. Medical reports are also analysed epidemiologically to provide data about ill-treatment in specific countries, and the quality of the final paper depends on the reliability of the original data.

The role of the medical profession in repressive states

The history of the medical profession at times of violent regimes taking power is a sad one. Medical organisations have often been key supporters of the totalitarian regime. In Nazi Germany, the medical profession needed to be reined back because it was indulging in eugenics to an extent that alarmed even the Nazi hierarchy.[30] In Chile, the Medical Association was instrumental in the strikes that helped bring down the elected Allende regime, and published lists of names of doctors who did not participate. After the coup, doctors pointed out to soldiers those colleagues who had supported the Allende regime, who were detained and sometimes executed.[31] However, five years later the Chilean Medical Association started organising human rights training and opposing the excesses of the regime. In the 1980s, the Medical Association of South Africa was quick to defend those doctors who were accused of human rights violations, and did not support those doctors who spoke out about torture.[23] Doctors have to prove that words about ethics are not just a way of evading external regulation, but are genuinely put into practice worldwide.

However, there are other good examples as well as the Chilean one. The Turkish Medical Association has done an enormous amount to protect prisoners and doctors. The hierarchy of the Syrian Medical Association was imprisoned *en masse* for protesting and never seen again.[32] The most important way of helping is to support openly those doctors who are being persecuted for criticising government policy on torture. As can be seen, such doctors do not always get the support they need from their national medical associations when they exist, and when the medical association supports such doctors, it comes under pressure from the government. Amnesty International, and particularly the Medical Network, is doing an excellent job of raising public awareness of doctors and other healthcare workers who are prisoners of conscience. This work needs to be extended, perhaps by the network organisations working together with the World Medical Association and other organisations, so that doctors who have come across cases of torture have a way of notifying it without necessarily putting themselves and their families at excessive risk. Official routes of complaint include the United Nations Committee Against Torture, the United Nations Special Rapporteur on Torture, and (in Europe) the European Committee for the Prevention of Torture.[9,28]

REFERENCES

1   Robertson AH, Merrills JG. Human Rights in the World. Manchester: Manchester University Press, 1996
2   Gillon R. Philosophical Medical Ethics. Chichester: John Wiley, 1985

3   Reyes H. Medical neutrality subject to National Law: should doctors always comply? Medcisch Contakt 1996; 51:1446–1460

4   Istanbul Protocol. See: Welsh J. The problem of torture, Chapter 1 in this book

5   Reyes H. The conflict between medical ethics and security measures. In: Gordon N, Marton R (eds), Torture. Human Rights, Medical Ethics and the Case of Israel. London: Zed Books, 1995, pp 41–47

6   Smidt-Nielsen K. The participation of health personnel in torture. Torture 1998; 8(3):91–94

7   British Medical Association. The Medical Profession and Human Rights: Handbook for a Changing Agenda. London: Zed Books, 2001

8   Principles of Medical Ethics relevant to the Role of Health Personnel, particularly Physicians, in the protection of Prisoners and detainees against Torture and Other Cruel, Inhuman or Degrading Treatment or Punishment. United Nations General Assembly resolution 37/194 of 18 December 1982

9   See: Welsh J. The problem of torture, Chapter 1 in this book

10 Selmouni v. France (Application No. 25803/94), Judgement of the European Court of Human Rights, Strasbourg, 28 July 1999

11 Body of Principles for the Protection of All Persons under Any Form of Detention or Imprisonment. United Nations General Assembly resolution 43/173 of 9 December 1988

12 Anonymous. Health care for prisoners: implications of 'Kalk's refusal'. Lancet 1991; 337:647–648

13 Iacopino V, Heisler M, Pishevar S, Kirshner RH. Physician complicity in misrepresentation and omission of evidence of torture in postdetention medical examinations in Turkey. JAMA 1996; 276(5):396–402

14 Reyes H. Medical and ethical aspects of hunger strikes in custody and the issue of torture. In: Oehmichen M (ed.), Maltreatment and Torture. Verlas Schmid-Roemhild: Luebeck, 1998

15 Peel M. Hunger strikes. BMJ 1997; 315:829–830

16 Johnnes Weir Foundation for Health and Human Rights. Assistance in Hunger Strikes: A Manual for Physicians and Other Health Personnel Dealing with Hunger Strikes. Amersfoort, JWFHHR: 1995

17 World Medical Association, Declaration of Malta, 1992

18 Standard Minimum Rules for the Treatment of Prisoners. Approved by the United Nations Economic and Social Council 31 July 1957 (resolution 663 C I (XXIV))

19 See, e.g., Report to the Finnish Government on the visit to Finland carried out by the European Committee for the Prevention of Torture and Inhuman or Degrading Treatment or Punishment (CPT) from 7 to 17 June 1998 (CPT/Inf (99) 9)

20 Vesti P, Somnier FE. Doctor involvement in torture. A historical perspective. Torture 1994; 4(3):82–89

21 Smidt-Nielsen K. Doctors involved in torture. Torture 1994; 4(1):9–10

22 Lopez JP, Aguilar AS, Castro MCR, Eleazar JG, McDonald A, Schweickart AP Doctors at risk. Torture 1996; 6(1):13–16

23 Welsh J. The role of codes of medical ethics in the prevention of torture. In: Gordon N, Marton R (eds), Torture. Human Rights, Medical Ethics and the Case of Israel. London: Zed Books, 1995, pp 48–62

24 Munro R. Judicial psychiatry in China and its political abuses. Columbia J Asian Law 2000; 14:1–128

25 See: Reyes H. Visits to prisoners and documentation of torture, Chapter 5 in this book

26 British Medical Association, Medicine Betrayed. London: Zed Books, 1992, pp 54–55

27 World Medical Association, Declaration of Tokyo, 1975

28 Giffard G, The Torture Reporting Handbook. Colchester: Human Rights Centre, University of Essex, 2000

29 See: Frey B. Documenting a well-founded fear: how medical caregivers can assist torture survivors in the asylum process, Chapter 3 in this book

30 Hanakauske-Abel HM. Not a slippery slope or sudden subversion: German medicine and National Socialism in 1933. BMJ 1996; 313:1453–1463

31 Waitzkin H, Modell H. Medicine, socialism, and totalitarianism: lessons from Chile. NEJM 1974; 291:171–177

32 Amnesty International. Forgotten victims: health professionals imprisoned in 1980, Syria. London: AI Index: MDE 24/06/95, 19 June 1995

5

VISITS TO PRISONERS AND DOCUMENTATION OF TORTURE

Hernan Reyes

The documentation of torture covers a wide range of situations that require different strategies. According to the context and circumstances involved, the type of interview and the procedures for getting documentation will vary considerably.[1] From the torture victim's point of view, there will be variations in perception, and adaptation to the situation, according to where and when the interview takes place. It cannot be stressed often enough that a humane approach towards, and true empathy for, the persons interviewed are more important from a humanitarian point of view than getting the actual documentation[2] – a paramount and sometimes neglected feature that workers in this field sometimes tend to forget.

Today there are dozens of major centres – and many more smaller ones – around the world that provide care for victims of torture. Some of these centres are in the countries where torture actually takes place; others are in host countries where victims of torture may perhaps seek asylum. Trained personnel with the necessary medical and psychological skills will obtain documentation in such centres while at the same time providing therapy. Legal advisors and social workers will also be present thus to provide not only medical expertise but also legal advice and social assistance. In these centres, time limitations for interviews will not be a major limiting factor, and having a series of interviews will be the rule rather than the exception.

Documenting torture is a very different matter when the persons having been assaulted are still in custody, often in the hands of the very authorities responsible for torturing them. They are therefore still, and often extremely, vulnerable.[3-6] As visits to prisoners are becoming more and more widespread, by workers from different backgrounds and organizations, the following general considerations are given for precisely those situations where victims of torture are still not free, and are in such custody. In other words, the authorities who are still holding them are very much still in control of their welfare and security.

The relationship established between these persons, and visitors from the outside who are not in a position to release them, is very different from the doctor–patient relationship in a therapeutic centre. Getting information about torture in countries where it is practised does not necessarily have to be, and often cannot be, done inside the prisons. In such cases, it is often possible to obtain information about torture by interviewing released prisoners or refugees, and collect the necessary data.

Visiting prisoners held in countries where torture takes place is of course useful for obtaining documentation about torture. Visits to prisoners have, however, a broader objective. One of the aims of the visit will of course be to attempt to put a stop to the practice of torture, the main reason for seeking proper documentation. However, just as important, visitors from the outside will provide solace and comfort to the prisoners, by the personal contact in itself. The encounter with outsiders will often implicitly recognize the fact that these prisoners are in a 'special' situation and that they are not forgotten. More important, visitors from the outside will often be able to provide liaison between the prisoners and their family members. Whatever be the actual circumstances – and these will differ greatly between continents and countries – it is necessary, before 'rushing in' to visit prisoners, to first establish initial safeguards so the visit itself does not put anyone in danger, and then to know which pitfalls to avoid during the actual visits.

Documenting torture should never become an objective absolute in itself. The *sine qua non* principle to keep constantly in mind is the same one that regulates all medical practice: 'above all do no harm'. Visits to prisoners are not objectives in themselves either, and should never become counter-productive for those persons visited, not even in the overall interest of documenting and combating torture.

Within the many scenarios possible, the main issue is thus the 'risk factor' for those persons to be interviewed. Visiting prisoners can sometimes put them in danger of reprisals, or of further abuse and torture, because what the prisoners may or may not have told the visitors during the visit may not please their custodians. This possibility has to be weighed before even thinking about getting access to persons in custody. Unless the visitors are certain they can guarantee the safety of all persons whom they interview, they should not take the risk of putting vulnerable prisoners in danger of reprisals. Once access to prisoners has been granted, and guarantees given, it shall be necessary to know about a series of pitfalls regarding working methodology and procedures, that will have to be avoided. In all contexts where torture is a major issue, the core question of potential risk to the persons visited should be constantly kept in mind, and re-evaluated as the need arises during the visit.

A clear distinction must be made between situations in which the torture victim is free to speak about his or her ordeal and feels safe to do so, and the situation where the torture victim objectively or subjectively fears reprisals for mentioning torture.

The first case may be, for example, a person having been tortured and seeking help from a specialist. This may mean medical help from a doctor, or legal help from a lawyer. There is no danger of him or her suffering any reprisal or coercion.

The second case is typically an interview with persons still in the custody of those very authorities who may have been responsible for inflicting torture. This may be in a prison, interrogation centre, or simply in a place where the torture victims have good reason to fear their oppressors may torture them again.

Documentation of torture will be very different in these two situations.

Box 5.1

Another aspect of this risk factor has to be considered when visiting prisoners. As has been stated, it is certainly not the aim of the visitors to cause any harm to the persons being interviewed, and the interviewees should not be putting themselves in danger of reprisals of any kind. In a less literal but no less important sense, victims of torture should never be forced to 'relive' their torture experience by having to tell their stories to the interviewers, i.e. to undergo 'retraumatization' during the documentation of torture. When visiting persons still in custody and potentially still in danger, the risk of opening a 'Pandora's Box' of retraumatization is very real. However qualified the visitor may be, the circumstances of such visits in no way resemble the therapeutic situation in the safety of an outside centre. This most important aspect of working with victims of torture is addressed specifically elsewhere.[7]

The following considerations on safeguards and pitfalls to avoid when visiting prisoners are based on years of institutional experience with the International Committee of the Red Cross (ICRC), working in countries around the world. ICRC teams visit prisoners in countries in conflict situations, ranging from outright war to civil disturbances or the aftermath of internal violence. The aim of such visits is not to seek the liberation of prisoners, but to see that they receive proper treatment and protection from any form of abuse, including torture, thereby safeguarding not only their physical and mental integrity but also their human dignity.

Visits to prisoners may not always involve contexts where torture is an issue. Admittedly, insalubrious and overcrowded prison conditions can be – and often are – used as a form of torture. For the purpose here, however, torture shall be considered in its more general definition, as in the 1984 UN Convention against Torture.

General safeguards for visits

Establishing trust between interviewer and interviewee

Using information obtained: respecting informed choice

Benefits of the visit for the victims interviewed

Considerations about the interviewee

Considerations about the interviewer

Considerations about the interview

Working with and through interpreters

Gender issues and torture

Box 5.2

GENERAL SAFEGUARDS FOR VISITS

Visits to prisoners for the purpose of documenting torture demand certain non-negotiable conditions and guarantees; without which they should not be attempted, as they may in that case be not only useless, but also counter-productive, as they may put the persons interviewed in further danger.[8,9]

In order to carry out visits in a professional and objective manner, certain safeguards of procedure need to be observed, if torture is at stake. The issue of possible reprisals for those persons to be interviewed should never be shirked, nor should the safety of the persons interviewed be taken for granted. It should be made perfectly clear to the detaining authorities that all persons to be interviewed should be able to come forward freely without any threat of any kind made or even insinuated. The authorities should give the interviewers guarantees to this effect before they begin the visit. Needless to say, precautions should be taken so as to ensure that such 'fair play' is actually respected. It would be unacceptable to take it for granted that reprisals will never take place merely because assurances have been received from the detaining authority to this effect.

The keystone to any visit to prisoners is to be able to interview all persons concerned, and who freely accept to be interviewed, in conditions of safety and privacy. Information about living conditions in custody may be very sensitive, and prisoners may be understandably reluctant to reveal details that concern themselves or other persons, even to visitors from the outside. Information regarding torture is obviously even more sensitive. On a first visit to prisoners in a country where torture is an issue, outsiders should not take for granted that all prisoners will necessarily trust visitors! In some (admittedly rare) cases, custodial authorities have been known to organize 'sham' Red Cross visits,[10] completely with fake identity cards. All visitors need to be able to convincingly identify themselves to prisoners, and clearly explain the scope of their intended work.

How many prisoners to visit, and which ones to choose when there are a great number of them are questions that of course will depend entirely on the actual situations. There are no foolproof sampling techniques or methods in a torture situation. First of all prisoner populations are anything but homogenous, and more important, prisoners should be offered a chance to come forward and speak – in the privacy of the interview – according to the need. Prisoners in isolation for months and years will have a greater need of contacting visitors from the outside than prisoners who live together and are allowed visits. The articles cited in the bibliography for further reading give more details on how visits to prisoners are actually organized.

Perhaps the key factor necessary for establishing trust between outside interviewers and prisoner interviewees will be the perceived and actual privacy of the interviews that actually take place in the prison setting. As will be developed further on, this usually means interviews without any interference from the authorities – meaning the prison hierarchy, guards, prison doctor and psychologist, etc. Experience has shown that, despite promises made to the visitors, detaining authorities often 'coach' prisoners as to what they can or cannot say to visitors. It is only through the safeguard of having interviews in private, that prisoners may decide it is safe for them to speak freely and divulge information about torture. In other cases, prisoners will desire privacy for personal reasons, as, understandably, torture can raise a series of very intimate matters that prisoners will want to keep private. In many cases, and this will be developed further on, the doctor(s) on the team will be the one(s) who need to expand the interview and offer the intimacy of the doctor–patient relationship and medical examination.

The confidentiality of the information received also has to be established in relation to fellow prisoners. As shall be mentioned further on, prisoners should also be protected from possible harm from other prisoners, and therefore the privacy of the interview should be unqualified. This key principle of interviews in private has therefore to be accepted by all, as a preliminary condition for interviewing prisoners.

Another key point has to be developed here concerning possible reprisals. The only way to ensure that prisoners are not subjected to harassment or outright reprisals for having talked to outsiders is to see and interview them again. Any and all prisoner(s) who potentially put themselves in danger by such interviews should be seen again. The interval between the first and second visit obviously will depend on the actual risk of foul play from the side of the detaining authorities. This may mean coming back the next week, or perhaps only some months late if the risk is small. It is in this sense that a 'one-shot' visit may be useless and even cause more harm than any good.[8] If prisoners are re-interrogated by their gaolers and suffer reprisals for what they may have said, the visit has possibly done more harm (for those individuals) than any good obtained from the information obtained.

It should therefore be evident that repeat visits to individuals, and not just to institutions, are necessary to ensure the safety of all prisoners interviewed who are potentially at risk for retaliation. In order to effectively be able to locate each person and personally (again, in privacy) interview him or her about any such reprisals, it is necessary to have some way of localizing each individual. This will need some system for taking down personal information so as to ensure reliable identification of the individuals concerned.

Registering identities of the people to be interviewed may not be a straightforward task. A method is required so as to ensure all information taken by a team is comparable and reliable. The authorities may agree to interviews but not necessarily to the taking down and confidential storing of personal information about prisoners. If a visit is only to a small group of well-known persons, the taking down of identities may not be imperative. If a large group of prisoners is visited – and is to be repeatedly visited – it will be necessary to address this issue.

One visit can be worse than no visits at all, if the personal security of the persons visited cannot be guaranteed.

Box 5.3

These safeguards – always repeating the visits, and ensuring a way of identifying the individuals who may need protection from reprisals – should be fully understood before undertaking any visits in contexts where torture is an issue. Even when such guarantees are obtained, there are no entirely foolproof safeguards. There will always exist the possibility of authorities going back on a promise to allow a repeat visit after the first one has already taken place. There may even be dire circumstances when it may be necessary to visit prisoners without the interviewers being absolutely sure of being able to see the persons they talk to again. Any such exceptions should be justi-fied by extraordinary circumstances, and be, precisely, exceptions recognized as such. Visiting teams should be accountable for any harm they may cause, and irresponsible 'visits' offering no guarantees should be discouraged.

In conclusion, one visit alone may provide information about torture, but will provide no safeguard to those prisoners who have put their trust in the interviewers. It would be unethical to obtain information about torture 'at any price', endangering the very people who have been tortured and who confide in the visiting team. The attitude 'one cannot make an omelette without breaking some eggs' is not acceptable when the personal safety of persons having put their faith in a visiting team is at stake.

ESTABLISHING TRUST BETWEEN INTERVIEWER AND INTERVIEWEE

When interviewing and examining prisoners about torture, it will be necessary to be able to talk to individuals in private. Useful and reliable information can only be obtained, however, if there is a relationship of trust between the prisoners and the interviewers. This fact is not 'self-evident' to the prisoners any more than it is to the authorities that authorize the visit. During the initial stages of the visit, it should be explained to the prisoners very clearly and exactly what the aims, objectives – and limitations – of the visit are, and what the procedure is to be for interviews. Most important, the time available should be clearly announced, and all dispositions taken so as to ensure a fair amount of time for each group of prisoners.[8] The procedure of the interview in private has also to be explained, and the fact that any information obtained during an interview in private will not be released to the authorities – indeed to anyone without the expressly given consent of the prisoner.

Group interviews during visits are useful for obtaining information on general condi-tions of imprisonment, or details about 'safe subjects' such as the food, access to the outside or availability of reading materials. Even these apparently 'innocent' subjects may be highly touchy – particularly when there are internal 'clans' or hierarchies amongst the prisoners themselves, often with internal coercion. Torture, however, by its very nature will most often be a subject that prisoners do not broach easily. The torture experience is also a very personal issue, and interviewers should not take for granted that prisoners already have spoken about it to fellow prisoners or even to family members during visits. Also, torture involves the infliction of humiliating and degrading practices, which most people have great difficulties speaking about. The privacy of the interview, and reassurance about the confidentiality of all aspects of the information received from the interviewee, has to be recalled at all times if one is to obtain any information at all.

Interviews about torture should thus be ensured strict privacy, as the element of trust is essential if one is to obtain reliable information about torture. This may be more easily said than done. One should obviously never conduct an interview in front of or within earshot of prison guards – however, even asking apparently innocent questions in the presence of custodial staff may be misinterpreted by the prisoners and make them wary of the interviewer. Even if the staff are not likely to report anything, prisoners may not feel comfortable if privacy is not strictly respected.

As has been said, privacy also means interviewing individuals without the presence of fellow inmates. Prisons are notorious for having 'collaborators' infiltrated into every group of prisoners. Prisoners themselves also often have internal hierarchies and rival clans. Torture may or may not be an issue between these groups, but there will be cases where internal pressures from amongst the prisoners will come to bear. Coercion and reprisals do not always come from the detaining authorities. Great care should be taken to protect those prisoners who have been tortured from any form of coercion. For this reason, it is most often not advisable to have interviews about torture in groups and for the prisoners' safety; the principle should be to have individual interviews, if torture is the issue at hand.

Interviewers should be firm on the principle of having talks in private when they visit prisoners and torture is the main issue at hand.

Box 5.4

In the same way that the trust of the detaining authorities may have to be won initially, when obtaining authorization for the visits, the prisoners themselves will often have to be persuaded to accept the 'legitimacy' of the visiting team. Prisoners may understandably be reluctant to put themselves in danger. The purpose of the visit will have to be duly – and convincingly – explained, and reassurances given about what will be done with any information received during the visit. It should not be forgotten that in any prison there are also 'agents provocateurs' amongst the prisoners themselves. These sometimes may goad inexperienced visitors into openly making statements about torture that may compromise the security of other prisoners or even jeopardize the visit itself. Also, it should not be forgotten that prisoners might inadvertently put themselves into danger in such situations. Interviewers should always be wary and take all necessary precautions, such as refusing to engage in open debates with groups of prisoners on topics that might put them in danger.

During a first visit, when prisoners and visitors do not as yet know each other, two diametrically opposite situations can arise. In one situation, prisoners may understandably not be willing to come forward, and may be too frightened to say anything, either about themselves or about torture – even when there are clearly visible signs of torture on their bodies. In this case, the visit will have to proceed slowly, and the interviewers explain clearly about the objectives and the limitations of the visit. If the prisoners are fearful of reprisals, and unless there is a rock-solid guarantee from the detaining authorities as to being allowed to repeat the visit, it may be best in some cases to not broach the subject of torture at all. Prisoners may be too afraid to even ask for interviews in private, as they may fear that by doing so they are 'marked' by the authorities – and may be called up after the visit to be interrogated by the authorities as to what was said.

In another situation, the prisoners, happy to see someone from 'the outside world' may be a bit too confident about their personal safety, and take ill-considered risks. This may, for example, involve openly denouncing a specific guard, known for his brutality, or by making statements they would normally never make, that, if overheard, might put them in danger. Some prisoners may want to make an open statement about 'the situation'. In such cases it is best to recall to them that they should not put themselves at risk. There is no 'one-fits-all' solution to such problems. The bottom line must, however, always be ensuring the safety of the prisoners by keeping interviews about torture within the framework of the interviews in private. In some cases, it may even be necessary to interview all the prisoners, so as not to put any one group of individuals 'on the spot'. Proceeding in this way will encourage prisoners to speak more freely during interviews.

In those cases when prisoners are reluctant to speak out, a good way to lead the way to private interviews is to begin with 'group' interviews on general topics, and then proceed to the subject of 'health'. One of the interviewers at least should always be a doctor. It will normally be readily understood that medical interviews should be held in private. Enquiring about the health system and the individual's personal state of health may be the first step to talking about torture – which is arguably a procedure deleterious to health.

The privacy of the 'medical interview' may be in some cases the only possible way to obtain information about torture. It cannot be repeated often enough that any information thus obtained should only be used by the interviewers if – and only if – the interviewees have given their consent to it being used.[11]

There may also be cases where the vast majority of the prisoners have visible scars of brutal torture on their bodies, but all are reluctant to having anything said about it out of fear of reprisals. In such a case, it may sometimes be useful to conduct what is known as a 'sanitary inspection' of all prisoners in the courtyard, thereby making it possible for the visitors (particularly the doctor), to see all the prisoners, and observe and document at least the visible scars of torture. This can then be done in full view of all concerned. The authorities will inevitably know that such an inspection has taken place and will not have anyone to pinpoint as having 'talked about torture'. More to the point, the prisoners will feel confident that this is so.

USING THE INFORMATION OBTAINED: RESPECTING INFORMED CHOICE

Consent should be a *sine qua non* condition for using any of the information about torture provided by prisoners during interviews. Some prisoners may have good reasons for not wanting their names to be used in any documentation. Others may be overly confident, and inadvertently put their full trust in the examiners, who may or may not be in a position to actually guarantee their safety. Interviewers have to state clearly and intelligibly exactly what they intend to do with the information they receive from the prisoners they interview, and have to specifically request permission for its use. Prudence and common sense have to be employed in considering this whole issue.

Prisoners may refuse permission for their stories to be used, out of fear of reprisals, despite being informed of the guarantees obtained by the interviewers beforehand. Any such refusals must be respected, even if and when the interviewers feel they are groundless. This may mean not using certain testimonies until such a time when the prisoners feel less afraid. Whatever the situation, interviewers should respect that which has been agreed with the prisoners over any other considerations. Regarding sensitive subjects, such as sexual torture and assault, it is undeniable that if the strictest confidentiality is not guaranteed, the fear of 'leakage' of what is rightly considered 'intimate information', will hamper the interviews.[12,13]

There is also the opposite, admittedly rarer, case of prisoners absolutely wanting their stories to be used to document torture, and specifically stating they do not care about any possible consequences. Some well-meaning interviewers believe they should 'veto' such a request, if they feel the security of prisoners cannot be guaranteed. This praiseworthy attitude has, however, to be weighed against the fact that a prisoner fully aware of possible reprisals has the right to insist that the information provided be used, even with identity details provided, if this is his or her true desire. It would be wrong to 'betray' the trust of such prisoners, willing to take a risk in the pursuit of a higher ideal (such as combating torture), and not use their testimonies because the interviewer is afraid for their safety. In all cases, interviewer and prisoners should openly discuss the issue, and whatever has been promised to the prisoner should be respected. Betraying the trust of a prisoner is unacceptable, whatever the good intents of the interviewer.

BENEFITS OF THE VISIT FOR THE VICTIMS INTERVIEWED

The aim of visits to prisoners when documenting torture is the issue is to obtain concrete information about methods and circumstances of torture, and effects and durable sequelae of torture on the persons who have suffered it. This will allow outside bodies to exert influence upon the perpetrators, the ultimate aim being to put a stop to the practice of torture.

This is an aim in itself, and arguably a justifiable one. However, the objective of visits should not be only to document torture. Ideally there should be some benefit for those persons who are interviewed and examined as well, who have already undergone torture and for whom that reality can never be reversed. The liaison with family members outside has been mentioned. Other benefits may be small: only the satisfaction of knowing that the information given will be useful to help prevent others in the future suffering the same. There should, however, also be some direct benefit to the prisoners themselves.

The benefit of the visit to those victims of torture interviewed can be the fact that for a brief moment, they have access to someone from the outside with some medical and psychological expertise. They can therefore feel free to ask any questions they have about their bodies and minds and the effects of their traumatic torture experience.[2,8] Just getting answers to questions about possible long-term sequelae, or about the possibility of treatment once they are free, can certainly provide some comfort and advice. Treatment itself, other than what minimum treatment can possibly be administered on the spot, will normally not be an option. The visitors should, however, be in a position to request and obtain any medical treatment needed. Needless to say, permission from the victim should be obtained before making any such transactions with the detaining authorities.

CONSIDERATIONS ABOUT THE INTERVIEWEE

The way to document torture will vary considerably according to the person having been subjected to torture. An interview with a political activist or political prisoner will be very different from that with a simple farmer caught up in a war situation,[14] *a fortiori* from a very sensitive interview with a girl having been raped by her oppressors.

It cannot be repeated enough here that *empathy*, real and not merely formal and institutional, is a paramount condition for anyone working with victims of torture.

'Doing no harm' may mean, in some cases, putting down one's pen and paper and merely listening to the victim's story, in cases where direct and full attention is required and when it becomes obvious that the victim feels uncomfortable with what resembles an 'interrogation' ... Interviewers should never take the risk of enhancing the injuries of torture by uncalled for assertiveness or aggressive interviewing. The persons interviewed should never feel they are being *obliged* to talk about their torture experience.

In the same light, interviewers should not forget that each individual has his or her own story to tell. When visiting a large number of prisoners, it is easy for the interviewer to forget this. The prisoner who has been waiting for her interview all day, and who has, from the interviewer's point of view, 'nothing new' to tell, should never be brushed away with the attitude of 'I-have-heard-this-story-already' ... Each individual deserves the same amount of attention and empathy, whether or not the details of the torture experience have already been heard. It is a mistake to think that all prisoners who have been tortured have already told all the details of torture amongst themselves. In many cases talking about torture simply is not done, at least not about the intimate aspects of torture and its consequences. Torture is a very personal traumatization,[7] and often prisoners only reveal certain details to interviewers from the outside, but if and only if they are received with understanding and empathy.

Care should be taken to distinguish between the 'veteran' political prisoner, who may be more 'resistant' to torture and more willing to talk about it and answer specific questions, and the 'bystanders', caught up in a situation they are in no way prepared for, and who are understandably more traumatized. More care may be necessary in interviews with the latter category, as they have been totally unprepared for the trauma of torture and its effects. The particularly sensitive issue of rape and sexual torture is discussed further on.

CONSIDERATIONS ABOUT THE INTERVIEWER

Interviewers who visit prisoners and want to document torture should expect difficult interviews. Non-medical interviewers may often find it very difficult to cope with the stories they hear, and the understandable, often shattering, reactions of the people they interview. Even medical interviewers often find it difficult to bear hearing descriptions of torture situations and the anguish of the victims whom they often have little to offer besides a little on-the-spot empathy.

Interviewers should be well prepared for their tasks, and be knowledgeable about the outside circumstances in the country where they work. It can be vexing, even insulting, to victims of torture to have to explain the obvious in the middle of their narratives, to interviewers who have obviously not done their homework on the political, cultural and historical context pertaining to the victims. Interviewers should make themselves familiar with the specific objectives of torture within the given context,[4,6,15–17] as well as with the local methods used by the torturers and the coping mechanisms relevant to the culture at hand.

In a new situation, interviewers obviously cannot be expected to have advance knowledge about everything, but they should not lose their credibility by having to ask too obvious questions. This will mean preparing for the visit beforehand, and learning from previous workers, local experts and publications by reliable sources[18] – all the while keeping awake a spirit of objectivity, and not develop pre-conceived attitudes.

Torture victims may have difficulties telling their stories. This may be for a number of reasons – cultural or religious taboos, feelings of guilt and/or shame,[14] psychological defence mechanisms,[19] impairment of memory, and not the least being fear and distrust regarding the visitors. The informed interviewer will therefore need to guide the victim along ('guide' and not 'direct' ...) and determine which mechanism is in play so as to handle the difficulties. If it is important to have some knowledge about the context, it is even more important to listen to the interviewee. Being knowledge-able about context and background should not, however, lead to pre-conceived categorization of torture.[20,21] Interviewers should approach torture and its conse-quences as a whole, and not reduce the information received to groupings of methods and symptoms.

The question of whether doctors or 'lay' persons should document torture, is a moot issue. There is undoubtedly a role for investigators from different backgrounds. What is important is for different workers to know their limits and to complement each other's talents and know how.

A physician interviewing a torture victim will concentrate more on psychological and physical sequelae than a layperson.[22] As has been stated, a physician will be able to answer specific questions about the effects and sequelae of torture. Visits to prisoners should never be done without a physician on the team, even if precisely only for this reason.[21] A non-medical person versed in human rights law will conduct the inter-view differently, and may gather information perhaps more useful to ascertain a pattern of abuse by a specific authority, rather than dwell on inflicted injuries. In the same light, the torture victim will probably bring forth different information to the interviewer with a legal background than to the physician. Both have important roles to play.

Documentation of torture carried out by investigators seen by the victims as being partial to the authorities responsible for the torture – whatever their actual intrinsic integrity – will obviously not produce the same information as one carried out by out-side independent investigators. A prison doctor investigating torture, no matter how sincere, will not be perceived in the same way as an outside doctor asking the same questions.

CONSIDERATIONS ABOUT THE INTERVIEW

The information about torture obtained from the interview with the torture victim will obviously vary between contexts and according to the time elapsed since the torture actually took place. Specific signs and symptoms have been reviewed extensively in many publications about torture, a selection of which are offered for further reading in the bibliography of this chapter. Similarly, the 'torture interview' and its subtleties have been extensively reviewed. There are, however, certain 'core' elements of the torture interview that apply more specifically to interviews with prisoners.

The use of questionnaires when visiting prisoners is debatable. The humane aspect of the visit, which is the restoration of personal contact with the prisoner, will be diluted if not altogether lost, if the essential part of the interview is to be conducted through a written impersonal checklist. In addition, a questionnaire will be time consuming, and any such standardization of a phenomenon as complex as torture, furthermore assessed through interviews in a prison setting, will be of dubious relevance.

The first point to remember when interviewing prisoners is to have in mind at all times the context. The interviewee is still vulnerable – whether *objectively* so or merely *subjectively* matters little. The effect is the same – and will regulate the rapport established between interviewer and interviewee.

It goes without saying that documentation of torture – and even more so interviews of prisoners – should only be done by trained interviewers,[2] with specific knowledge about what they are doing and knowledgeable about the different methods and effects of torture. The purpose of the interview has to be explained clearly and in a vocabulary adapted to the level of comprehension of the interviewee, so as to encourage a frank and open relationship with interviewer. Establishing a relationship of trust may take time and be difficult. It may require more than one interview, and it is not rare to learn much more about torture concerning individuals on a second or third visit than on the initial interview.

The structuring of the interview will depend greatly on the context and on the personal situation of each interviewee. Obviously directed questions should be avoided ('Were you tortured when they arrested you?') in favour of open, general questions ('When you were arrested, how did it go?').[8]

Cultural norms should be taken into account, which may in some cases imply asking roundabout questions first, about family for example, before getting to the situation in the prison and the issue of actual torture. Elsewhere it might be considered impolite to ask about a prisoner's family before a rapport of trust has been established, and the objective of the visit and interview fully understood by the interviewee. There are no 'one-fits-all' methods for conducting interviews.

In the same light, interviewers, often apprehensive about 'forgetting something' sometimes use checklists. It holds true, perhaps even more so when interviewing about torture, that when one asks questions all one gets is answers... A checklist approach often intimidates the interviewee, who may even reduce his or her answers to nods of the head. Experience has also shown that some interviewers, content with having gone through the whole list, have in fact not identified some fact that should have been obvious just by looking at the interviewees, and letting them tell their story instead of 'grilling' them.

If on the one hand, directive interviews are to be avoided, on the other, leaving verbose interviewees free rein in what, of necessity in a prison situation, is a limited time period, may be totally counter-productive. This leads to the question of how much time is 'enough' time for a torture interview. Here circumstances and local customs will often dictate actual practice. In some countries, interviews will take one or two hours, in others there may be no more than 20–25 minutes available per person. Whatever the limit adopted for the needs of the visit, it will always be insufficient. This has to be announced to the prisoners in advance so as to avoid understandable frustration. It also has to be remembered that prisoners can and should be seen again during the next and following follow-up visits.

The questions to ask will vary greatly from context to context. Geographical details of where torture takes place may be easier for interviewees to remember than chronological specifications on how long any one method was applied. Chronology may not be in itself crucial to the issue at hand, as often it is difficult for a prisoner to determine the lapses of time. More important than such specifications, description of what happened and how it was perceived and 'what happened next' may be more relevant to the story.

Interviewers, with or without medical training, should know about the effect of 'potentialization'. Several methods of torture applied simultaneously with, for example, 'hooding' or 'blindfolding' can have greatly enhanced effects – more severe than one would expect from simply applying them together to the same person. This is particularly true for the psychological effects, for example of never being able to anticipate what direction a blow is coming from. Applying electrical current to someone suspended by the arms tied behind his back while blindfolded can provoke spasmodic contractions much more severe and painful than if the victim can see (and prepare himself for) the same torture. This is just one example to show that knowledge of the mechanisms of torture is necessary if the interviewer is to fully comprehend the victim's story. The 'unpredictable' and 'uncontrollable' aspects of torture have been studied extensively.[14,19]

A 'listing of methods' approach to documenting torture, meaning recording all the different forms of torture used by the oppressors, may be counter-productive if presented as such a 'catalogue' in a report. The clinical picture produced by torture first of all varies greatly between individuals, even more so between cultures and contexts. As has been stated, it is much more than the simple sum of effects produced by each of the methods listed. Such a 'package deal approach' to documentation of torture will inevitably reduce any dialogue with the alleged perpetrators to a discussion of which methods from the list qualify as torture and which do not – rather than a discussion on the prohibited use of torture in itself.[22,23]

It is now generally accepted that 'the worst scars are in the mind'.[23] It is, however, not futile to recall here that a 'WYSIWYG approach'[24] is not useful and indeed can be counter-productive. Physical torture obviously can leave scars, but interviewers should refrain from concentrating merely on physical scars. A solid and well re-structured description of torture should include, if useful, description of scars, but should not give the impression that their presence is the necessary 'proof' required for torture. Torturers have known for a long time how to minimize marks left on the body, and psychological torture, while it may indeed have physical effects, may leave no traces.

Torture methods involving third persons, particularly when family members are concerned, can be even more traumatic than torture to the person

'I didn't mind the pain so much. It was the cries next door I couldn't bear.'[25]

Thus when documenting torture, it should be kept in mind that inquiring merely about torture inflicted to the person can be misleading. In the same light, sham executions are extremely traumatic, but are sometimes neglected by interviewers. There is still insufficient knowledge about the mental and emotional consequences of torture. This is even more so regarding about transcultural differences in responses to torture. It may therefore make little sense to try to 'categorize' severity of torture, and to try, for example, to contrast sham executions, sexual assaults, solitary confinement and physical pain in overall comparative tables. In addition, an absence of certain symptom patterns, physical or psychological, in no way will mean that the interviewee did not experience torture. As is stated clearly in the Istanbul Protocol, 'Absence of Evidence is not Evidence of Absence'.[1]

Finally, interviewers should be aware of coping mechanisms used, unconsciously in most cases, by victims of torture. Torture victims will, for example, often have mentally blocked out the more painful memories of their torture experience, and it can be counter-productive to try to open up such recollections during interviews that are of necessity short and sketchy, and not followed up by professional help.

WORKING WITH AND THROUGH INTERPRETERS

Communication with victims of torture will sometimes be straightforward, when there is a common language between the investigator and the victim. Ideally, all interviewers should speak the language of the prisoners interviewed. This is unfortunately very often not a realistic possibility. In all other circumstances, the necessary 'middleman' will be the interpreter. Working with an interpreter presents specific difficulties when dealing with the issue of torture.[8,22,23]

The issues already mentioned, i.e. knowing about the historical, cultural and ethnic background of the victims, obviously also apply for interpreters. Some workers try to get around the cultural obstacles by using interpreters from the same local background as the victims. While this may be acceptable in a 'therapeutic centre' situation, it should best be avoided when visiting prisoners. Experience has time and again shown that it can be at the very least counter-productive, and sometimes dangerous for both interpreters and victims, as well as making what is already difficult enough a task even more so.

Local interpreters, no matter how devoted and trustworthy, may be putting themselves into dangerous situations by working with interviewers when documenting torture. Experience has shown that such interpreters can be put under pressure, either themselves or their families, by the authorities, to reveal information about interviews in which they have served as interpreters. Apart from putting the interpreters themselves in an uncomfortable situation, this also betrays the trust between interviewers and prisoners, and might even put the latter in danger as well.

Furthermore, in many situations, even when coercion by the authorities may not be an issue, using local interpreters can lead to mistrust by the prisoners themselves. What to think, for example during the Balkans conflicts of the nineties, of using interpreters from one specific ethnic group to visit prisoners from 'the opposite' ethnic group, in the custody of the same ethnic group as the interpreters. The interpreters could be put under pressure by the authorities, but more to the point, would not necessarily be trusted by the prisoners, no matter how reliable their own personal integrity. If interpreters from the same ethnic group as the prisoners were used, this could be to the liking of the prisoners (unless they were to be seen as 'collaborators' ...) but would possibly get them into trouble with the custodial authorities from the other group ... The same reasoning would obviously be identical whatever the nationalities in such a conflict.

It is therefore best policy never to use local interpreters but to rely on 'expatriate' ones. This may complicate (and make more expensive) the task at hand, but is a necessary condition if the work is to be done in a professional way. Disastrous situations have occurred through the use of local interpreters who turned out to be not as neutral as they appeared, or who were put under extreme pressure from malevolent influences. In the worst cases, naïve interviewers can be 'manipulated' by biased interpreters who interpret only part of the story – and who are simply not trusted by the prisoners they help interview.

Interpreters should ideally be professional one who know all the subtleties of the language, religion and culture of the persons interviewed – and not just expatriates who more or less speak the local language. Experience has shown that the choice of the interpreter goes well beyond merely speaking a language, and that the sensitivity rightly demanded of all who interview torture victims, need to be all the more present in the interpreters.

It should be fully realized that it is the interpreters who are on the 'front line' of the torture interview, which is why it is so important that cultural, religious and ethnic sensitivities be fully grasped beforehand. Only in this way will they be able to faithfully relay the information and convey the subtleties received. This is a key issue in documenting torture, as a lack of sensitivity from the interpreters can ruin any hope of interviewing prisoners and obtaining any information.

Working through interpreters is not always intuitive. One's natural tendency to look at the person speaking and being spoken to should be trumped when working with an interpreter. The interviewer should always look, not at the interpreter, but at the interviewee when presenting her or himself, and when asking questions. Likewise, when the prisoner answers or speaks for him or herself, it is the prisoner who should be observed, even if not a word is understood. Observing body language, gestures and facial expressions, as well as non-verbal communication is of paramount importance. Some words concerning known methods of torture will invariably be (or at least, should be) recognized (e.g. 'telefono', 'darmashakra', 'cheera', etc). Acknowledgement of such terms, even by just nodding, will show the interviewee that one is familiar with the local situation. The torture victims themselves will invariably talk to the interpreter, often at great lengths. This is quite normal and the interviewer should certainly not 'take offence' for what is an understandable reaction. However, the interviewer should not take this 'time out' to get his or her notes in order, but should on the contrary always look at the interviewee and somehow show him or her that the interviewer is giving full attention to the situation.

When the interpreter is not a trained professional, there is the risk of the interviewer 'losing control' of the interview. The torture victim may understandably get 'carried away' when talking to someone – the interpreter – who knows his or her language. A non-professional interpreter might also 'lead' the interview or 'launder' what the torture victim has to say according to pre-conceived opinions, modesty or even personal bias. Some information is inevitably lost during any translated interview, but this should be kept to a minimum, and outright distortions absolutely avoided. Interviewer and interpreter have to learn how to work together as a team. Sometimes a 'literal' (i.e. word-for-word) translation will be required. More often, the interpreter will have to provide as accurate a linguistic connection as possible between what involves two different cultures, all the while remaining as objective as possible.[1]

When preparing a visit to prisoners, it is necessary to compare notes with the interpreter beforehand, and exchange any notions of vocabulary that may come up during the interviews. Concerning medical terminology, if the interpreter is not knowledgeable about terms of anatomy or other system functions, the interviewer should explain what terms she or he expects to use, so as to limit awkward exchanges in front of the interviewee to a minimum. Interviewers should avoid esoteric words or internal 'jargon', so as to avoid misunderstandings (and quibbling) in front of the interviewee. Interpreters also need to be warned about the nature of the torture accounts they may hear, particularly if they are not used to working with torture victims, and need to be able to control their personal reactions. Their rendering of what is stated should not be distorted by their own emotional reactions.

It should always be taken into consideration that interpreters are priceless members of the team, and are often, in fact, the 'cultural consultants' for the team. Interpreters should be called on, after a day's work, to give their impressions of the situation. They who receive the prisoners' narratives directly, may have important pieces of information, whether or not related to torture directly, that may be crucial to comprehending the whole story. Good interpreters will point out and explain relevant cultural, historical and social factors and linguistic idioms to the interviewers, and the team will enrich its vocabulary accordingly as it goes along.

As a rule, 'fellow inmates' should not be used as interpreters, except for topics that cannot possibly put anyone in a difficult situation (e.g. explaining the workings of the septic tank in a prison should not necessarily need a professional expatriate interpreter). For interviews about torture, however, as for any other subject which is touchy and controversial, fellow prisoners should be avoided. As has been mentioned, prisoners have internal hierarchies and clan systems that are difficult to know about, and using a prisoner from one group to interpret for members of another can be dangerous. A 'too-willing' friendly interpreter from one cell might not be acceptable for the next cell. Inversely, a prisoner should never be asked to interpret for another one unless one is sure there is no problem.[8]

In some cases it will not be possible to find an independent expatriate interpreter, for example when some of the prisoners speak only dialects. In such cases, taking precautions so as not to put anyone into awkward situations or in danger, using the interpretation of a fellow inmate may be the only way to interview someone who shares no common language with the visiting team. The safest way is to make known to the prisoner to be interviewed that she or he should choose someone from his or her friends to translate what is being said. This may or may not work out, and at all times interviewers should be aware of the possible pitfalls. It may be best to pass up an interview rather than insist on having it at all costs and possibly create trouble for the prisoner.

Finally, the issue of confidentiality about the information received concerns interpreters possibly even more than interviewers, as they, of necessity, are the only ones to have the 'full story'. Interpreters should agree beforehand to respect confidentiality in the same terms as what is required of all interviewers.

GENDER ISSUES AND TORTURE

The issue of gender will have greater or lesser importance according to the context. In countries where men and women can exchange conversations without any hesitation, and where female doctors as well as male doctors work interchangeably with either gender, there should be less of a problem conducting interviews. This of course by no means rules out individual problems that may arise, as torture by its very nature is meant to humiliate and degrade those submitted to it. Furthermore, medical examinations may be simply out of the question, or at least very uncomfortable, when there is a gender difference between interviewer and interviewee. This applies even more particularly to all forms of sexual torture, or any torture targeting the genitals. Gender sensitivities need to be considered and taken into account in all contexts.[2]

In many of the countries where torture takes place, these gender issues are a serious barrier. For religious or cultural reasons – or both – men are often not supposed to address unmarried women directly, and often it is out of the question for a male doctor to approach a woman, let alone examine her unclothed in any circumstance. For such extreme cases, and indeed for most cases where cultural practices will frown upon men examining women and vice versa, it will be necessary to provide for interviewers, and even more important, physicians of both sexes. This may be a complication and involve additional difficulties and costs, but it would be inconsiderate to say the least to neglect interviewing female prisoners, for example, for want of a woman doctor when documenting torture. In the same light, in many countries where torture of males targets the genitals specifically, to even consider documenting such torture through a female physician (or assisted by a female interpreter!) should be unthinkable.

This being said, a parenthesis is warranted here. Apart from the obvious culturally extreme cases, there may be times when the function of the interviewer is intrinsically more important than his or her gender. For example, in a case where women have been raped and are afraid of being pregnant, or are fearful for their future fertility, it may be more important for them to be able to ask questions to a male doctor, who is best equipped to provide answers, than to speak to a female interviewer who is not a physician and cannot give any reassurance.[14] In some cases, it may be possible to find compromise solutions, with 'chaperones' present for interviews or medical examinations. Ideally, however, gender should be respected, and interviewing teams should provide for professionals from both sexes.

CONCLUSION

Documenting torture in situations where the victims of torture are still in the custody of those same authorities allegedly responsible for torturing them is very different from interviewing torture victims in the calm and reassuring setting of a therapeutic centre. Specific precautions have to be taken, to ensure the safety and security of the persons to be interviewed, when they are therefore potentially vulnerable. Safeguards need to be considered so that no person interviewed is subjected to reprisals for having spoken to the visitors. Promises and guarantees need to be supplemented with actual means of control to ensure there is no foul play. This may involve being able to trace individual prisoners who were or felt themselves to be, at risk for reprisals or punishments.

Above all, however, it should never be forgotten that visits to prisoners who have been or may have been tortured first of all need to be compassionate and carried out with genuine empathy. Interviewers should not let their eagerness for information lead them to neglect the humane aspect of their rapport with those persons interviewed. Care must be taken not to open 'Pandora's boxes' that cannot be closed.

Interviewers need to create a climate of trust with the prisoners they interview. This is not easy and implies that the interviewers must be clear in explaining their objectives and limitations, and that they respect the confidentiality they must guarantee to all those who speak with them. Any information entrusted to them must only be used if the interviewers have obtained the full consent of those concerned.

Physicians are an indispensable part of the team, as they are able to provide specific answers to the many questions that will be asked by then victims of torture. This specific assistance and counsel will perhaps be the only concrete 'benefit' the interviewers will give to the persons they see during a visit.

Transcultural differences must be fully appreciated by the interviewers before they begin to work with prisoners. This is particularly important if they have to work through interpreters, who should also observe confidentiality and work in a professional way.

Gender differences must be respected, and both interviewers and interpreters should be of both genders so as to respect any cultural sensitivities. As this will also prevent any loss of information in cases of sexual torture or generally when conducting medical examinations during assessment.

REFERENCES

1   Chapter V, General interview considerations. In: Istanbul Protocol (see: Welsh J. The problem of torture, Chapter 1 in this book)
2   Daudin P, Reyes H. How visits by the ICRC can help prisoners cope with the effects of traumatic stress. In: Danieli Y, Rodley N, Weisaeth L (eds), International Responses to Traumatic Stress. Amityville: Baywood Publishing Company, 1996, pp 219–256
3   Reyes H. The conflict between medical ethics and security measures. In: Gordon N, Marton R (eds), Torture. Human Rights, Medical Ethics and the Case of Israel. London: Zed Books, 1995, pp 41–47
4   British Medical Association. Medicine Betrayed. London: Zed Books, 1992

5   Cassese A. Inhuman States: Imprisonment, Detention and Torture in Europe Today. Cambridge: Polity Press, 1996

6   Iacopino V. Torture in Turkey and its Unwilling Accomplices. Boston: Physicians for Human Rights, 1996

7   Chapter VII, Psychological evidence of torture. In: Istanbul Protocol (see: Welsh J. The problem of torture, Chapter 1 in this book)

8   Reyes H. Visits to prisoners by the ICRC. Torture Supplementum No. 1 1997, 28–30

9   Reyes H. Visits to prisoners: International Committee of the Red Cross at work. Torture 1993; 3(2):58

10 Personal communication to the author by ICRC delegates in the field

11 In some cases, reports to governmental authorities will contain the actual identities (with the consent of all concerned) of the victims making allegations of torture. In other cases, only general statements will be made, without anyone being identifiable. In *all* cases, consent must be sought beforehand and clearly marked on the individual files drawn up during the interviews

12 In many (most?) cultures, the shame and stigma around sexual assault is such that torture victims outside prison will often prefer not to go near a treatment center – which could make people suppose they might have been raped – rather than seek advice or help, even if such information is desperately needed

13 Skylv G. The nature of human experience: some interfaces between Anthropology and Psychiatry. Lecture at the Royal Society of Medicine, London, 1992

14 Paker M, Paker O, Yuksel S. Psychological effects of torture: an empirical study of tortured and non-tortured non-political prisoners. In: Basoglu M (ed.), Torture and its Consequences. Cambridge: CUP, 1992, pp 72–82

15 Stover E, Nightingale E. The Breaking of Bodies and Minds. New York: WH Freeman, 1985

16 Suedfeld P. Psychology and Torture. New York: Hemisphere Publications, 1990

17 Peter Taylor. Beating the Terrorists: Interrogation in Omagh, Gough and Castlereagh. New York: Penguin Books, 1990

18 Amnesty International. Stamp Out Torture. London: AI Publications, 2000

19 Basoglu M, Mineka S. The role of uncontrollable and unpredictable stress in post-traumatic stress responses in torture survivors'. In: Basoglu M (ed.), Torture and its Consequences. Cambridge: CUP, 1992, pp 182–226

20 Reyes H. Torture and its consequences. Torture 1995; 5(4):72–76

21 Staiff M. Visits to detained torture victims. Torture 2000; 10(1):4–7

22 Doctors examining victims of torture will have a very different role to play according to the task they are to accomplish. A physician acting as a medical examiner will not have the same approach as a physician acting in a therapeutic role, or as an independent examiner for an NGO

23 Personal communication, Professor Sten Jakobsen, Karolinska Institute, Stockholm

24 'What you see is what you get', meaning concentrating on those visible scars of torture, giving the obviously erroneous impression that torture that leaves no scars is somehow 'less important' ...

25 Quoted in Basoglu M (ed.), Torture and its Consequences. Cambridge: CUP, 1992

6

HISTORY TAKING

Vincent Iacopino

INTRODUCTION

The primary purpose of obtaining historical information from an individual alleging torture or ill treatment is to elicit a narrative account from which to assess physical and psychological evidence of torture or ill treatment. However, history taking is important for a number of other reasons. Before interviewing subjects, clinicians should be aware of the purposes that history taking may serve:

- *Narrative account:* The narrative account provides subjective information that may be cross-referenced with objective findings such as those observed on the physical/psychological examination and/or legal documents. Subjective historical information may, of course, be cross-referenced with other historical information provided in the narrative. For example, one may be able to assess the degree of consistency between descriptions of torture methods/restraint techniques and allegations of subsequent injuries.

- *Historical evidence of torture:* Although physical and psychological findings of torture and ill treatment may be regarded as important confirmatory evidence that a person was tortured, such acts of violence against persons frequently leave no marks or permanent scars. Therefore, the absence of such evidence should not be construed to suggest that torture did not occur. Historical information such as descriptions of torture devices, body positions and methods of restraint, descriptions of acute and chronic wounds and disabilities, and identifying information about perpetrators and the place(s) of detention may be very useful in corroborating an applicant's allegations of torture. Historical evidence of torture or ill treatment may be corroborated internally within an individual's narrative account and/or may be corroborated externally by accounts of others' torture. In order to assess for corroborating historical information between individuals, it may be useful for clinicians to develop databases from individuals they have evaluated from specific regions. Such databases may not be practical or useful until the clinician has interviewed a considerable number of subjects from the same country/region.

- *Dynamic process of interpretation:* The clinician's interpretation of findings actually begins in the process of asking questions. It is a dynamic process of inquiry that is increasingly informed by the subject's responses to both the clinician's questions and what the clinician learns from the content of the narrative account. In the course of taking the history, the clinician may begin to assess the degree of consistency of the information provided. Since the credibility of the subject is often an issue in medical–legal cases in which torture and/or ill treatment is alleged, it is important for the clinician to pursue any and all inconsistencies that may be present in an individual's narrative account. Inconsistencies may be categorized as either internal or external. For example, an internal consistency may arise when a subject is able to describe torture devices and/or perpetrators, but had previously indicated that he/she was blind-folded. An external inconsistency may exist when an account of torture is not supported by many other accounts of torture from the same region. Under such circumstances, the most prudent course of action is to first suspend judgment and pursue possible clarifications. In the absence of an adequate clarification with additional questioning, it may be advisable to present the inconsistency to the subject directly and provide the opportunity for clarification. Persistent inconsistencies should be interpreted in the context of all evidence in the case and should be communicated to the subject's legal counsel as well.

- *Developing trust:* Trust is an essential component of eliciting an accurate account of abuse. The process of eliciting the history represents the opportunity to earn the subject's trust. Earning the trust of one who has experienced torture and other forms of abuse requires active listening, meticulous communication, courteousness and genuine empathy and honesty. Clinicians must have the capacity to create a climate of trust in which disclosure of crucial, though per-haps very painful or shameful, facts can occur. Important here is the awareness that those facts are sometimes intimate secrets that the person may reveal at that moment for the first time. In addition to providing a comfortable setting, adequate time for the interviews, refreshments and access to toilet facilities, the clinicians should explain what the patient can expect in the evaluation. The clinician should be mindful of the tone, phrasing and sequencing of questions. (Sensitive questions should be asked only after some degree of rapport has developed.) Also, the clinician should acknowledge the patient's ability to take a break if needed or to choose not to respond to any question he or she may not wish to.

- *Therapeutic intervention:* Although the clinician may elicit historical informa-tion primarily to document evidence of torture and ill treatment, the process of providing a narrative account of abuse often carries therapeutic implications. Communicating traumatic experiences may enable individuals to begin to process the meaning and the emotional pain of their experiences. As men-tioned above, the clinician's assessment may represent the first time that the subject has shared his/her traumatic experiences. While the recounting of traumatic events can have therapeutic value, it is important for clinicians to anticipate the possibility of re-traumatization.[1] For this reason, the examining clinician needs to assess the subject for possible clinical follow-up.

INTERVIEW CONSIDERATIONS

Before eliciting historical information, the clinician should be aware of a number of considerations that may affect the quality and accuracy of medical evaluations. Some of these considerations are discussed elsewhere in this book,[1] such as the use of interpreters, gender issues, interviewing in detention settings and re-traumatization. Additional factors include: the setting and timing of the interview, the clinician's approach to the subject, communication barriers, the level of detail and variability in the history, preparation for the interview, and qualifications of the examining clinician.

Interview setting and timing

The location of the interview and examination should be as safe and comfortable as possible. A two to four hour interview time may not be sufficient enough to conduct an evaluation for either physical or psychological evidence of torture. Furthermore, at any given time that an evaluation is conducted, situation-specific variables such as the dynamics of the interview, feelings of powerlessness in the face of having one's intimacy intruded upon, fear of future persecution, shame about the events, and survivor guilt may simulate circumstances of a torture experience. This may enhance the patient's anxiety and increase his/her resistance to disclosure of relevant information. A second, and possibly a third interview, may need to be scheduled to complete the evaluation.

In addition, the individual needs to be given the opportunity to request breaks, interrupt the interview at any time, and be able to leave if the stress level becomes intolerable, with the option of a consecutive appointment. Access to refreshments and toilet facilities should be provided as well.

Clinician's approach to the subject

Establishing rapport with the subject is essential for conducting an effective and complete evaluation. The clinician should introduce the interview process in a manner that explains in detail the procedures to be followed (questions asked about medical psychosocial history including history of torture and current physical and psychological functioning) and that prepares the individual for the difficult emotional reactions that the questions may elicit. The clinician should acknowledge the patient's ability to take a break if needed or to choose not to respond to any question he/she may not wish to. Priorities should be negotiated. For example, issues regarding time limitations should be clarified.

Clinicians need to be sensitive and empathic in their questioning while remaining objective in their clinical assessment. At the same time the interviewer should be aware of potential personal reactions to the survivor and the descriptions of torture that might influence the interviewers perceptions and judgments. The interview process may remind the survivor of being interrogated during torture. Therefore, strong negative feelings toward the clinician may be evoked such as fear, rage, revulsion, helplessness, confusion, panic, hatred, etc. The clinician should allow for the expression and explanation of such feelings, and express understanding for the individual's difficult predicament.

In addition, the clinician's responses to working with victims of torture and ill treatment (countertransference) may compromise the effectiveness of the medical evaluation. Common countertransference issues include: disillusionment, avoidance, withdrawal, helplessness, hopelessness, over-identification, idealization, anger, guilt, and loss of perspective. The clinician may experience symptoms of 'vicarious traumatization' such as nightmares, anxiety, and fearfulness over hearing the experiences told to them. Considering survivors' extreme vulnerability and propensity to reexperience their trauma when it is either recognized or treated, it is critical that health providers maintain a clear perspective of a healing relationship. Effective documentation of torture and other forms of ill treatment requires significant understanding of the motivations for working in this area. It is important that a clinician not use the population to work out unresolved issues in himself/herself, as these issues can clearly get in the way of effectiveness.

Communication barriers

The clinician should also try to anticipate, and when possible, address possible barriers to effective communication. Barriers to communication can drastically influence the value and/or process of an interview. Possible barriers to communication include:

- Environmental barriers such as lack of privacy, comfort of interview setting, inadequate time for the interview.

- Physical barriers such as pain or other discomfort the individual may be experiencing as a result of his/her abuse: for example, physical pain, difficulty sitting for extended periods, fatigue, sensory deficits such as blindness or deafness.

- Psychological barriers such as fear/anxiety, mental health disorders such as depression, posttraumatic stress disorder, or cognitive deficits.

- Sociocultural barriers such as the gender of interviewer (this is particularly important with victims of sexual assault), and language issues including appropriateness and accuracy of interpreter.

Level of detail in the history

In the course of obtaining a narrative account of events and experiences, the clinician should attempt to obtain as much detail as possible. So-called 'thick narratives' often provide more information from which to assess correlations between allegations and findings and frequently provide a sense of 'being there' that adjudicators often consider supportive of the individual's credibility. However, the inclusion of detailed historical information may be considered irrelevant by some adjudicators. Furthermore, attempts to obtain a detailed history may elicit accounts of events and experiences of which individuals are less certain. Also, when an individual has difficulties with memory and concentration, it is possible that a detailed history may conflict with earlier testimony. For this reason, it is important to inform the subject at the start of the interview of the importance of providing detailed information of only those events/experiences for which he/she has a reasonable degree of certainty.

Variability in the history

It is important to keep in mind that there is often variability in the amount and detail of information that an individual will recall with regards to the events of the trauma. This is often the case when an individual was subjected to repeated episodes of torture and/or ill-treatment. Furthermore, individuals may have been detained under conditions in which they lose a sense of time and/or place, for example, being kept blindfolded or held in solitary confinement in a dark cell, or were in a very weakened state as a result of being deprived of food, water or sleep. Furthermore, interviewers should use judgment about how much specific detail is needed to document the alleged abuse. For example, if someone was repeatedly tortured or raped, it is not necessary, nor perhaps appropriate, to try and elicit all of the details about every single episode.

Memory for events can be affected in one or more of at least three ways:[2]

- A failure to lay down memory (e.g. head injury, extreme emotional arousal).

- The motivated forgetting of unpleasant memories.

- Impaired ability to recall (e.g. severe depression).

There is also variability with regards to the degree of physical and psychological signs, symptoms or consequences which a survivor of torture and/or ill-treatment will manifest. Similarly, there is variability in the manner in which survivors of torture conduct themselves in interviews in recounting the events of their abuse. For example, some survivors may react with great emotion and frequently become tearful. Others may appear extremely calm or detached, describing the events as if they had happened to someone else.

Preparation for the interview

In preparation for the interview, it is useful to review appropriate documents and affidavits that the subject's legal counsel may have prepared. Such documents may help the clinician to anticipate the content of the individual's narrative and/or possible examination findings. Also, knowledge of prior testimonies may aid in identifying inconsistencies in the history. Despite the utility of legal documents and affidavits, the information contained therein should not be relied upon. All information relevant to a medical evaluation should be gathered by the clinician.

Preparing for an interview with a person alleging torture and/or ill treatment may seem to be an overwhelming experience when clinicians have limited understandings of the culture, ethnicity, religion, political landscape, etc. of the subject being interviewed. Clinicians have a responsibility to understand the context within which abuses such as torture occur. Also, regional practices of torture and ill treatment and their consequences are particularly relevant for clinicians. Such background information is often available in human rights reports by UN and non-governmental organizations. Discussions with colleagues who may have additional regional knowledge and expertise may help in preparing for the interview. Even clinicians who have accumulated considerable experience in conducting medical evaluations in specific regions may be confronted with knowledge deficits in the course of an evaluation, i.e. the cultural significance of a particular act. Under such circumstances, experienced and inexperienced clinicians alike, should seek clarification from the interviewee and/or the interpreter.

Given the emotional difficulties associated with the recounting of traumatic experiences, individuals may not show up for his/her appointment. Establishing contact just prior to the appointment can help prevent the frustration and inefficiency of missed appointments.

Clinician qualifications

Medical evaluations should be conducted by licensed clinicians. An individual's primary symptoms and findings and the availability of examiners often determines whether the examination is conducted by a medical doctor, such as a primary care physician, a specialist, and/or a mental health professional.

Assessments of physical and psychological evidence of torture and ill treatment may be conducted by one or more clinicians depending on their qualifications. With adequate training, a physician may qualify as an expert on both physical and psychological evidence of torture. For example, it is certainly appropriate for a primary care physician to evaluate physical findings as well as common mental health problems such as anxiety and depression. Whenever possible, interviewers should be prepared to comment on both the physical and psychological findings.

Medical evaluations of asylum applicants should be conducted with objectivity and impartiality. The evaluations should be based on the health professional's clinical expertise and professional experience. The ethical obligation of beneficence demands uncompromising accuracy and impartiality in order to establish and maintain professional credibility.

When possible, clinicians conducting medical evaluations should have specific essential training in forensic documentation of torture and other forms of physical and psychological abuse. They should have knowledge of prison conditions and torture methods used in the particular region where the patient was imprisoned, and the common aftereffects of torture. Physicians for Human Rights as well as other medical and human rights organizations sponsor training on methods of documenting torture.

TECHNIQUES OF QUESTIONING

Several basic rules must be respected during the interview:

- Information is certainly important, but the person being interviewed is more so.

- Listening is more important than asking questions. If you only ask questions, all you get is answers.

- To a torture survivor, it may be more important to talk about family than to talk about torture. This should be duly considered, and time allowed for some discussion of personal matters.

- Torture, particularly sexual torture, is a very intimate subject, and may not come up before a follow-up visit – or even later. Individuals should not be 'forced' to talk about any form of torture if they feel uncomfortable about it.

Structure inquiries to elicit a chronological account of the events experienced. Whenever possible, one should utilize open-ended questions (e.g. Can you tell me what happened? or Tell me more about that) and allow the individual to tell his/her story with as few interruptions as possible. This may result in a more accurate and detailed disclosure of information than moving too quickly to a rapid-fire form of questioning, which may, in fact mimic interrogation. Further details can be elicited with appropriate follow-up questions.

Leading questions should be avoided wherever possible in interviewing for medico-legal purposes, as the testimony could then be challenged in court. Closed questions and particularly list questions can cause confusion in the patient and might create unnecessary inconsistencies. For example, a man might be asked 'were you arrested by the police or the army?' If he were arrested by a special task force of soldiers and policemen working together, he would find it difficult to give an accurate answer without appearing to contradict the doctor.

Some questions may need some explanation in the asking, especially when the question lacks a cultural foundation or there is a serious social stigma associated with the individual's response (e.g. sexual assault). In such cases, the question may be phrased as follows: 'People who have memory problems or bad dreams have often been tortured or traumatized. Is this something that has happened to you?' In the case of sexual assault: 'People who have been detained are sometimes abused sexually, is this something that has happened to you?' Most often, individuals who have been tortured will respond with relief that you know that such things occur and that you are able to treat such matters seriously. However, in a medico-legal report it should be clear that answers were to potentially leading questions, and should be described, for example, as: 'On direct questioning, Mr X said that ...'

It is important for the clinician to bear in mind that torture survivors may have difficulty recounting the specific details of the torture for several important reasons, including

- factors during torture itself such as blindfolding, drugging, lapses of consciousness, etc.;

- fear of placing oneself or others at risk;

- lack of trust for the examining clinician and/or interpreter;

- psychological impact of torture and trauma such as high emotional arousal, and impaired memory secondary to trauma-related mental illnesses such as depression and posttraumatic stress disorder;

- disorientation and/or lapses in consciousness;

- neuropsychiatric memory impairment from beatings to the head, suffocation, near drowning, and starvation;

- protective coping mechanisms such as denial and avoidance;

- culturally prescribed sanctions that allow traumatic experiences to be revealed only in highly confidential settings.[3]

Inconsistencies in a person's story may arise from any or all of these factors. If possible, the clinician should ask for further clarification. When this is not possible, the clinician should look for other evidence that supports or refutes the story. A network of consistent supporting details can corroborate and clarify the person's story. Although the individual may not be able to provide the details desired by the clinician such as dates, times, frequencies, exact identities of perpetrators, etc., overall themes of the traumatic events and torture should emerge and stand up over time.

TAKING THE HISTORY[4]

Clinicians should not assume that the individual, such as the asylum applicant's attorney, requesting a medical–legal evaluation has related all the material facts. It is the clinician's responsibility to discover and report upon any material findings that he/she considers relevant, even if they may be considered irrelevant or adverse to the case of the party requesting the medical examination. Findings that are consistent with torture or other forms of ill treatment must not be excluded from a medical–legal report under any circumstance.

At the outset of the interview, the clinician should establish the identity of the subject and introduce him/herself. Law enforcement officials should not be present during the evaluation. If such officials refuse to leave the examination room, it should be noted in the clinician's report and/or the evaluation may be cancelled.

Psychosocial history – pre-arrest

The examiner should inquire into the person's daily life, relations with friends and family, work/school, occupation, interests, and use of alcohol and drugs, prior to the traumatic events. Inquiries into prior political activities and beliefs and opinions are relevant insofar as they help to explain why the person was detained and/or tortured, but such inquiries are best made indirectly by asking the person what accusations were made, or why they think they were detained and tortured. The psychosocial history is particularly important in understanding the meaning that individuals assign to traumatic experiences.

Past medical history

Obtain a complete medical history, including prior medical, surgical and/or psychiatric problems. Be sure to document any history of injuries before the period of detention and any possible after-effects. Knowledge of prior injuries may help to differentiate scars related to torture from those that are not.

Summary of detention(s) and abuse

Before obtaining a detailed account of events, elicit summary information, including dates, places, duration of detention, frequency and duration of torture sessions. A summary will help to make effective use of time. In some cases where survivors have been tortured on multiple occasions, they may be able to recall what happened to them, but often cannot recall exactly where and when each event occurred. In such circumstances, it may be advisable to elicit the historical account by methods of abuse rather than as a series of events during specific arrests.

Similarly, in taking a history it may often be useful to have 'what happened where' documented as much as possible. 'Holding places' are often operated by different security/police/armed forces, and what events happened in different places may be useful to get a full picture of the torture system. Obtaining a map of where the torture occurred may be useful in piecing together different histories from different people. This will often prove very useful for the overall evaluation.

Circumstances of detention(s)

Consider the following questions: What time was it? Where were you? What were you doing? Who was there? Describe the appearance of those who detained you. Were they military or civilian, in uniforms or in plain clothes? What type of weapons were they carrying? What was said? Were there any witnesses? Was this a formal arrest, administrative detention, or disappearance? Was violence used, threat spoken? Was there any interaction with family members? Note the use of restraints or blindfold, means of transportation, destination, and names of officials, if known.

Prison/detention place conditions

Include access to and descriptions of food and drink, toilet facilities, lighting, temperature, ventilation. Also, document any contact with family, lawyers or health professionals, conditions of overcrowding or solitary confinement, dimensions of the detention place, and whether there are other people who can corroborate his/her detention. Consider the following questions: What happened first? Where were you taken? Was there an identification process (personal information recorded, fingerprints, photographs)? Were you asked to sign anything? Describe the conditions of the cell/room (note size, others present, light, ventilation, temperature, presence of insects, rodents, bedding, and access to food, water and toilet). What did you hear, see and smell? Did you have any contact with people outside, or access to medical care? What was the physical layout of the place where you were detained?

Methods of torture and ill treatment

In obtaining historical information on torture and ill treatment, one should be cautious about suggesting forms of abuse that a person may have been subjected to. This may help to separate potential embellishment from valid experiences. However, eliciting negative responses to questions about various forms of torture also may help to establish the credibility of the person.

Questions should be designed to elicit a coherent narrative account. Consider the following questions: Where did the abuse take place, when and for how long? Could you see? Why not? Before discussing forms of abuse, note who was present (give names, positions). Describe the room/place. What objects did you observe? If possible, describe each instrument of torture in detail; for electrical torture, the current, device, and number and shape of electrodes. Ask about clothing/disrobing/change of clothing. Record quotations of what was said during interrogation, insults to one's identity, etc. What was said among the perpetrators?

For each form of abuse note: body position/restraint, nature of contact, including duration, frequency, anatomical location, and the area of the body affected. Was there any bleeding, head trauma, or loss of consciousness? Was the loss of consciousness due to head trauma, asphyxiation, or pain. One should also ask about how the person was at the end of the 'session.' Could he/she walk? Did she/he have to be helped back or carried back to the cell? Could he/she get up the next day? How long did the feet stay swollen? All this gives a certain completeness to the description, which a 'checklist' of methods does not.

The history should include the date(s) of positional torture, how many times and for how many days the torture lasted, the period of each episode, the style of the suspension (reverse-linear, being covered by thick cloth-blanket, etc., or being tied directly by a rope, putting weight on the legs or pulling down), or other position, etc.

In suspension torture, ask what sort of material was used (rope, wire and cloth leave different marks (if any) on the skin after suspension). The examiner must remember that statements of the length of the torture session by the torture survivor are subjective, and may not be correct, since disorientation of time and place during torture is a generally observed finding.

Was the person sexually assaulted in any manner? Elicit what was said during the torture. For example, during electric shock torture to the genitals perpetrators often tell their torture victims that they will no longer have normal sexual function, or something similar.

The distinction between physical and psychological methods is artificial. For example, sexual torture generally causes both physical and psychological symptoms, even when there has not been any physical assault. This list of torture methods provided below is given to show some of the categories of abuse possible. It is not meant to be used by clinicians as a 'checklist', nor as a model for listing torture methods in a report. A method-listing approach may be counterproductive, as the entire clinical picture produced by torture is much more than the simple sum of lesions produced by methods on a list. Torture methods to consider include, but are not limited to:

1   blunt trauma: punch, kick, slap, whips, wires, truncheons, falling down;

2   positional torture: suspension, stretching limbs apart, prolonged constraint of movement, forced positioning;

3   burns: cigarettes, heated instrument, scalding liquid, caustic substance;

4   electric shock;

5   asphyxiation: wet and dry methods, drowning, smothering, choking, chemicals;

6   crush injuries: smashing fingers, heavy roller to thighs/back;

7   penetrating injuries: stab and gunshot wounds, wires under nails;

8   chemical exposures: salt, chili, gasoline, etc. (in wounds, body cavities);

9   sexual: violence to genitals, molestation, instrumentation, rape;

10   crush injury or traumatic removal of digits and limbs;

11   medical: amputation of digits or limbs, surgical removal of organs;

12   pharmacologic torture: toxic doses of sedatives, neuroleptics, paralytics, etc.;

13   conditions of detention, e.g.:

 • small or overcrowded cell,

 • solitary confinement,

- unhygienic conditions,

- no access to toilet facilities,

- irregular and/or contaminated food and water,

- exposure to extremes of temperature,

- denial of privacy,

- forced nakedness;

14 deprivations:

- of normal sensory stimulation, such as sound, light, sense of time via hooding, isolation, manipulating brightness of the cell,

- of physiological needs: restriction of sleep, food, water, toilet facilities, bathing, motor activities, medical care,

- of social contacts: isolation within prison, loss of contact with outside world – victims often are kept in isolation in order to prevent bonding and mutual identification and to encourage traumatic bonding with the torturer;

15 humiliations: verbal abuse, performance of humiliating acts;

16 threats: of death, harm to family, further torture and/or imprisonment, mock executions;

17 threats to or arranging conditions for attacks by animals such as dogs, cats, rats, and scorpions;

18 psychological techniques to break down the individual: forced 'betrayals', learned helplessness exposure to ambiguous situations and/or contradictory messages, etc.;

19 violation of taboos;

20 behavioral coercion:

- forced to engage in practices against one's religion (e.g. forcing Muslims to eat pork),

- forced to harm others: e.g. the torture of others, or other abuses,

- forced to destroy property,

- forced to betray someone placing them at risk for harm;

21 forced to witness torture or atrocities being inflicted on others.

Review of symptoms

Obtain a detailed review of physical and psychological symptoms and disabilities at the time of the abuse and subsequently, up to the present time. All complaints of the torture survivor are of significance; although there may or may not be a correlation with the physical findings, they should be reported. Acute and chronic symptoms and disabilities associated with specific forms of abuse and the subsequent healing processes should be documented.

Acute symptoms

The individual should be asked to describe any injuries that may have resulted from the specific methods of alleged abuse. For example, bleeding, bruising, swelling, open wounds, lacerations, fractures, dislocations, joint stress, hemoptysis, pneumothorax, tympanic membrane perforation, genitourinary system injuries, burns (color, bulla, necrosis according to the degree of burn), electrical injuries (size and number of lesions, their color and surface characteristics), chemical injuries (color, signs of necrosis), pain, numbness, constipation, vomiting, etc. The intensity, frequency and duration of each symptom should be noted. The development of any subsequent skin lesions should be described and whether or not they left scars. Ask about health on release; was he/she able to walk, confined to bed? If confined, for how long? How long did wounds take to heal? Were they infected? What treatment was received? Was it a doctor or a traditional healer? Note the individual's ability to make such observations may have been compromised by the torture itself or its after-effects and should be documented.

Chronic symptoms

Elicit information of physical ailments that the individual believes were associated with torture or ill treatment. Note the severity, frequency and duration of each symptom and any associated disability or need for medical and/or psychological care. Even if the after-effects of acute lesions may not be observed months or years later, some physical findings may still remain, such as electrical current or thermal burn scars, skeletal deformities, malunion of fractures, dental injuries, loss of hair, and myofibrosis. Common somatic complaints include headache, back pain, gastrointestinal symptoms, sexual dysfunction, muscle pain, and common psychological symptoms include depressive affect, anxiety, insomnia, nightmares, flashbacks and memory difficulties.[5]

Psychosocial history (post-arrest)

Obtain information concerning the individual's post-detention/torture psychosocial history, including any difficulties the individual may have experienced such as continued harassment or persecution by authorities, fear for his/her own safety as well as the safety of family/friends following release from detention, inability to return to work or school. Obtain summary information concerning the events of the individual fleeing his/her country of origin and arrival in subsequent locations.

REFERENCES

1   See: Reyes H. Visits to prisons and documentation of torture, Chapter 7 in this book
2   Stone JH, Roberts M, O'Grady J, Taylor OV. Faulk's Basic Forensic Psychiatry. Oxford: Blackwell, 2000
3   Mollica, Caspi-Yavin. Overview: the assessment and diagnosis of torture events and symptoms. In: Başoğlu M (ed.), Torture and its Consequences, Current Treatment Approaches. Cambridge: Cambridge University Press, 1992, pp 38–55
4   Material in this section is excerpted from Iacopino V, Rosoff R, Heisler M. Torture in Turkey and its Unwilling Accomplices. Boston: Physicians for Human Rights, 1996, pp 221–231; and The Istanbul Protocol (see: Welsh J. The problem of torture, Chapter 1 in this book)
5   See: Allden K. The psychological consequences of torture, Chapter 7 in this book

7

THE PSYCHOLOGICAL
CONSEQUENCES OF TORTURE

Kathleen Allden

INTRODUCTION

Psychological reactions to torture present physicians, clinicians, and social scientists with the challenge of evaluating and assisting individuals who have survived crises of life threatening proportions. For many that have survived torture, the experience can cause profound effects at a deeply personal level that can persist and fluctuate for many years.[1,2] Psychological consequences develop in the context of personal meaning and personality development. They will vary over time and are shaped by cultural, social, political, interpersonal, biological, and intrapsychic factors that are unique for each individual. One should not assume that all forms of torture have the same outcome. However, over the past two decades much has been learned about psychological, biological, and neuropsychiatric responses to extreme stress including torture and clusters of typical symptoms have emerged that are recognized across cultures.[3] This chapter sets a framework for the evaluation and documentation of the psychological impact of torture that is mindful of these considerations.

The United Nations Convention Against Torture of 1984 defines torture as

' ... any act by which severe pain or suffering, whether physical or mental, is intentionally inflicted on a person for such purposes as obtaining from him or a third person information or a confession, punishing him for an act he or a third person has committed or is suspected of having committed, or intimidating or coercing him or a third person for any reason based on discrimination of any kind, when such pain or suffering is inflicted by or at the instigation of or with the consent or acquiescence of a public official or other person acting in an official capacity. It does not include pain or suffering arising only from, inherent in or incidental to lawful sanctions.'[4]

The World Medical Association in the Declaration of Tokyo (1975) interprets torture more broadly. In this declaration, torture is defined as 'the deliberate, systematic or wanton infliction of physical or mental suffering by one or more persons acting alone or on the orders of any authority, to force another person to yield information, to make a confession, or for any other reason.'[5] Both definitions of torture acknowledge that mental suffering is often the intention of the torturer. Since World War II, there has been much scientific investigation concerning the consequences of severe psychological trauma, including torture. As one of the editors of Istanbul Protocol,[6] this author will present the challenges relevant to developing the international standards for psychological assessment of survivors of torture, as well as pertinent information about evaluation, diagnosis and documentation of the psychological and social impact of torture and severe forms of human rights abuse.

THE PARADOX OF PSYCHOLOGICAL CONSEQUENCES OF TORTURE

The psychological consequences of torture present two paradoxes. First, psychological wounds are the most personal, intimate, and enduring consequences of torture and can affect not only the victim but also his/her family and community. Yet these scars are invisible; there are no objective signs, measurable parameters, lab tests or X-rays that document psychological wounds. The goal of torture is not to simply physically incapacitate the victim, but to reduce the individual to a position of extreme helplessness and distress and break his/her will.[7,8] At the same time, torture sets horrific examples to those that come in contact with the victim[9] and can profoundly damage intimate relationships between spouses, parents and children, and other family members, as well as relationships between the victims and their communities. In this way, torture can break or damage the will and coherence of entire communities.

The second paradox is that despite the fact that torture is an extraordinary life experience capable of causing a wide range of psychological suffering, extreme trauma such as torture does not always produce psychological problems. Therefore, if an individual does not have mental problems, it does not mean that he/she was not tortured. When there are no physical or psychological findings, this does not refute or support whether torture actually occurred.

SOCIAL, POLITICAL, AND CULTURAL CONTEXT

There are three complementary approaches for understanding the psychological impact of torture. The personal approach is the individual's story as told through testimony, oral history, literature, and art. The clinical approach utilizes a medical and psychological paradigm and relies on clinical history, physical exam, and mental status exam. The community approach involves epidemiological studies of traumatized groups and populations. In combination these approaches provide a broad and deep understanding of the impact of torture on human beings. Each approach requires consideration of the context of torture. Torture has unique cultural, social, and political meanings for each individual. These meanings will influence an individual's ability to describe and speak about their experiences. Similarly, these factors contribute to the impact that the torture inflicts psychologically and socially. Cross-cultural research reveals that phenomenological or descriptive methods are the best approaches when attempting to evaluate psychological or psychiatric reactions and disorders because what is considered disordered behaviour or a disease in one culture may not be viewed as pathological in another.[10-12] WHO's multi-centre cross-cultural study of depression conducted in the 1980s[13] provides a helpful guiding principle. That is, while some symptoms may be present across differing cultures, they may not be the symptoms that concern the individual the most. Therefore, the clinician's inquiry has to include the individual's beliefs about their experiences and meanings of their symptoms, as well as an evaluating the presence or absence of symptoms of trauma-related mental disorders.

Torture is powerful enough on its own to produce mental and emotional consequences, regardless of the individual's pre-torture psychological status.[14] Nevertheless, torture has variable effects[15] on people because the social, cultural, and political contexts vary widely.[16,17] Outcomes can be influenced by many interrelated factors that include but are not limited to the following:

- circumstances, severity and duration of the torture;

- cultural meaning of torture/trauma and cultural meaning of symptoms;

- age and developmental phase of the victim;

- genetic and biological vulnerabilities of the victim;

- perception and interpretation of torture by the victim;

- the social context before, during, and after the torture;

- community values and attitudes;

- political factors;

- prior history of trauma;

- pre-existing personality.[6]

For example, the consequences are different for a young woman who is raped during torture and is from a culture that attaches a severe negative stigma of impurity to a woman who has been raped, compared with a former military officer who is captured and suffers long-term solitary confinement and multiple beatings. It goes without saying that both types of torture are extremely severe, yet the impact on the individual's life is vastly different. The young woman might be socially ostracized and condemned even by her own family and community. The former military officer may have brain damage from beatings to the head with resultant long-term disability.

SELF-REPORT AND THE CONTROVERSY ABOUT TRAUMATIC MEMORY

Self-reports of trauma and torture are often not believed or felt to be distortions or exaggerations for purposes of obtaining asylum, compensation or other benefits and secondary gain. Self-reported physical and psychological symptoms are often construed as fabrications or exaggerations for the same reasons. This is reflected in the scepticism many refugees and asylum seekers encounter when confronted by government officials and others in authority. Much recent neuropsychological research has focused on memory distortion, reconstructing the past, and psychological trauma.[18] Some studies suggest that with increased psychological symptoms there will be exaggerations of traumatic events.[19] Other studies document a direct dose effect between exposure to trauma and level of psychological symptomatology.[20,21]

Contributing to this puzzle are descriptive clinical reports that reveal complaints of cognitive disturbances among diverse traumatized groups.[22] Research about survivors of prisoner of war camps and concentration camps reveals neurocognitive deficits and suggest that physical insults, particularly starvation, vitamin deficiency, and beatings to the head are major contributing factors.[23–25] Certainly, it is often under-recognized that many torture survivors have been subjected to physical injury to the brain from beatings to the head, suffocation, near drowning and severe, prolonged nutritional deficiencies and that these insults may lead to cognitive impairment in torture survivors.[2,26]

Complicating the picture even more is the finding that depression[27] and posttraumatic stress disorder (PTSD)[28] affect cognition. There are multiple hypotheses about why this may be true ranging from alterations in neuroendocrine systems,[29] to neurotoxic effects of severe stress on hippocampal neurons,[30] to psychoanalytic mechanisms.[31] Memory impairment as a result of these factors may affect the accuracy of the details a survivor is asked to provide about his/her torture. Despite these potential limitations, it is often of critical importance for a torture survivor to provide accurate details of his/her torture and trauma experiences because these details will be used in legal affidavits for political asylum, human rights investigations, and other legal and judicial purposes such as war crimes tribunals. The inability to produce detailed and precise recollections about dates, times, places, environmental descriptions, and descriptions of perpetrators can reflect negatively on the survivor's credibility and lead to severely deleterious consequences such as deportation of the survivor back to an extremely dangerous home country, denial of family reunification, prolonged detention, or failure to produce evidence to convict war criminals. Because of these grave outcomes, the clinician must take extra care to put the survivor's trauma history, clinical history, mental status examination and physical examination together with knowledge of the political context of the country where the torture allegedly took place, cultural idioms and beliefs, and social customs and barriers to full disclosure of traumatic events. The clinician must attempt to obtain as complete picture as possible of the individual's life experiences and the context in which they were experienced in order to speak to the credibility of the story and the believability of the clinical symptomatology.

RISK FACTORS, AND NATURAL HISTORY OF TRAUMA- AND TORTURE-RELATED DISORDERS

Despite the variability due to personal, cultural, social, and political factors, certain psychological symptoms and clusters of symptoms have been observed among survivors of torture and other types of violence.[3] Since 1980, the diagnosis of PTSD[32] has been applied to an increasingly broad array of individuals suffering from the impact of widely varying types of violence. Although the utility of this diagnosis in non-Western cultural groups has not been clearly established, evidence suggests that there are high rates of PTSD and depression symptoms among traumatized refugee populations from multiple different ethnic and cultural backgrounds.[20,33–36]

The core symptoms and signs of severe trauma and torture across cultures have become increasingly clear.[37] Many are physiological reactions that can persist for years. The main psychiatric disorders associated with torture are PTSD and Major Depression.[13] One does not have to be tortured to develop PTSD and/or Major Depression because these disorders appear in the general population. Similarly, everyone who has been tortured does not develop PTSD and Major Depression.

The course of Major Depression and PTSD varies over time. There can be asymptomatic intervals, recurrent episodes, and episodes during which an individual is extremely symptomatic. Therefore, when conducting an evaluation of a torture survivor, one must consider the following questions: (1) What is the timeframe of onset of symptoms; did symptoms occur immediately following the traumatic events or were they delayed for weeks, months, or even years? (2) Is there a history of recurring episodes of symptomatology? (3) How do problems and symptoms emerge over time? (4) Where is the survivor in the recovery process at the time of the assessment?

In considering who may be at heightened risk for developing psychological problems, one must evaluate both general/overall risk factors as well as those risk factors specific to traumatized populations including how trauma affects family and social relationships and other natural supports. The general risk factors for developing mental illness are based on age, sex, education, social class, divorced/widowed status, history of mental illness, and family history of mental illness. Additional risk factors for torture survivors include torture, war, political oppression, imprisonment, witnessing or experiencing atrocities, loss of family and/or separation from family, and distortion of social relationships. If the torture survivor is also a refugee or asylum seeker, he/she has the further risk factors of migration (loss of home, loved ones, possessions, etc.), acculturation, poverty, prejudice, cultural beliefs and traditional roles, cultural and linguistic isolation, absence of adequate support systems, and unemployment or underemployment. The multiple layers of increasing risk present a clinical picture that has been described by as one of 'cumulative synergistic adversity.'[38]

CONDUCTING THE PSYCHOLOGICAL EVALUATION

Psychological evaluations may take place in a variety of settings and contexts resulting in important differences in the manner in which evaluations should be conducted and in the way symptoms are interpreted. For example, whether or not certain sensitive questions can be asked safely will depend on the degree to which confidentiality and security can be assured. An evaluation by a clinician visiting a prison or detention centre may be very brief and not allow for as detailed an evaluation as one performed in a clinic or private office that may take place over several sessions and last for several hours. At times some symptoms and behaviours typically viewed as pathological may be viewed as adaptive or predictable, depending on the context. For example, diminished interest in activities, feelings of detachment and estrangement would be understandable findings in a person in solitary confinement. Likewise, hypervigilance and avoidance behaviours may be necessary for those living under threat in repressive societies.[39]

The clinician should attempt to understand mental suffering in the context of the survivor's circumstances, beliefs, and cultural norms rather than rush to diagnose and classify. Awareness of culture specific syndromes and native language-bound idioms of distress is of paramount importance for conducting the interview and formulating the clinical impression and conclusion. When the interviewer has little or no knowledge about the victim's language and culture, the assistance of an interpreter is essential. An interpreter from the victim's country of origin will facilitate an understanding of the language, customs, religious traditions, and other beliefs that will need to be considered during the evaluation.

Clinicians should be aware of the potential emotional reactions that evaluations may elicit in survivors. Fear, shame, rage, and guilt are typical reactions. A clinical interview may induce mistrust on the part of the torture survivor and possibly remind him or her of previous interrogations thereby 'retraumatizing' him or her. To reduce the effects of retraumatization, the clinician should communicate a sense of empathy and understanding. The victim may suspect the clinician of having voyeuristic and sadistic motivations or may have prejudices towards the clinician because he/she has not been tortured. The clinician is a person in a position of authority and for that reason may not be trusted with certain aspects of the trauma history. Alternatively, individuals still in custody may be too trusting in situations where the clinician cannot guarantee that there will be no reprisals for speaking about torture. Torture victims may fear that information that is revealed in the context of an evaluation cannot be safely kept from being accessed by persecuting governments. Fear and mistrust may be particularly strong in cases where physicians or other health workers were participants in the torture. In the context of evaluations conducted for legal purposes, the necessary attention to details and the precise questioning about history is easily perceived as a sign of doubt on the part of the examiner. Under these pressures, survivors may feel overwhelmed with memories and affect or mobilize strong defences such as withdrawal and affective flattening or numbing during evaluations.

If the gender of the clinician and the torturer is the same, the interview situation may be perceived as resembling the torture more than if the genders were different. For example, a woman who was raped and tortured in prison by a male guard is likely to experience more distress, mistrust, and fear when facing a male clinician than she might experience with a female. On the other hand, it may be much more important to the survivor that the interviewer is a physician regardless of gender so as to ask specific medical questions about possible pregnancy, ability conceive later, and future of sexual relations between spouses.

When listening to individuals speak of their torture clinicians should expect to have personal reactions and emotional responses themselves. Understanding these personal reactions is crucial because they can have an impact on one's ability to evaluate and address the physical and psychological consequences of torture. Reactions may include avoidance and defensive indifference in reaction to being exposed to disturbing material, disillusionment, helplessness, and hopelessness that may lead to symptoms of depression or 'vicarious traumatization', grandiosity or feeling that one is the last hope for the survivor's recovery and well-being, feelings of insecurity in one's professional skills in the face of extreme suffering, guilt over not sharing the torture survivor's experience, or even anger when the clinician experiences doubt about the truth of the alleged torture history and the individual stands to benefit from an evaluation.

PSYCHOLOGICAL FINDINGS AND DIAGNOSTIC CONSIDERATIONS

It is prudent for clinicians to become familiar with the most commonly diagnosed disorders among trauma and torture survivors and to understand that it is not uncommon for more than one mental disorder to be present as there is considerable co-morbidity among trauma-related mental disorders. The two most common classification systems are the International Classification of Disease (ICD-10)[40] Classification of Mental and Behavioral Disorders and the Diagnostic and Statistical Manual of the American Psychiatric Association-Edition IV (DSM-IV).[32] Non-mental health clinicians such as internists and general practitioners that perform evaluations of torture survivors should be familiar with the common psychological responses to torture and be able to describe their clinical findings. They should be prepared to offer a psychiatric diagnosis if the case is not complicated. A psychiatrist or psychologist skilled in the differential diagnosis of mental disorders related to severe trauma will be needed for particularly emotional individuals, cases involving multiple symptoms or atypical symptom complexes, psychosis, or in cases presenting confusing clinical pictures.

The diagnosis most commonly associated with torture is PTSD. Typical symptoms of PTSD include re-experiencing the trauma, avoidance and emotional numbing, and hyperarousal. Re-experiencing can take several forms: intrusive memories, flashbacks (the subjective sense that the traumatic event is happening all over again), recurrent nightmares, and distress at exposure to cues that symbolize or resemble the trauma. Avoidance and emotional numbing include avoidance of thoughts, conversations, activities, places, or people that arouse recollection of the trauma, feelings of detachment and estrangement from others, inability to recall an important aspect of the trauma, and a foreshortened sense of the future. Symptoms of hyperarousal include difficulty falling or staying asleep, irritability or outbursts of anger, difficulty concentrating, hypervigilance, and exaggerated startle response.

Depressive states are almost ubiquitous among survivors of torture. Depressive disorders may occur as a single episode or be recurrent. They can present with or without psychotic features. Symptoms of Major Depression include depressed mood, anhedonia (markedly diminished interest or pleasure in activities), appetite disturbance, insomnia or hypersomnia, psychomotor agitation or retardation, fatigue and loss of energy, feelings of worthlessness and excessive guilt, difficulty concentrating, and thoughts of death, suicidal ideation, or suicide attempts.

A survivor of severe trauma such as torture may experience dissociation or depersonalization. Dissociation is a disruption in the integration of consciousness, self-perception, memory and actions. A person may be cut off or unaware of certain actions or may feel split in two and feel as if observing him or herself from a distance. Depersonalization is feeling detached from oneself or one's body.

Somatic symptoms such as pain and headache, and other physical complaints, with or without objective findings, are common problems among torture victims. Pain may shift in location and vary in intensity. Somatic symptoms can be directly due to physical consequences of torture, be of psychological origin, or both. Also, various types of sexual dysfunction are not uncommon among survivors of torture particularly, but not exclusively, among those who have suffered sexual torture or rape.

Psychotic symptoms may be present such as delusions, paranoia, hallucinations (auditory, visual, olfactory, or tactile), bizarre ideation, illusions, or perceptual distortions. Cultural and linguistic differences may be confused with psychotic symptoms. Before labelling someone as psychotic, one must evaluate the symptoms within the individual's cultural context. Psychotic reactions may be brief or prolonged. It is not uncommon for torture victims to report occasionally hearing screams, his or her name being called, or seeing shadows, but not have florid signs or symptoms of psychosis. Individuals with a past history of mental illness such as bipolar disorder, recurrent major depression with psychotic features, schizophrenia and schizoaffective disorder may experience an episode of that disorder.

The ICD-10 includes the diagnosis 'Enduring Personality Change'. PTSD may precede this type of personality change. To make the ICD-10 diagnosis of enduring personality change, the following criteria must have been present for at least two years and must not have existed prior to the traumatic event or events. These criteria are hostile or distrustful attitude towards the world, social withdrawal, feelings of emptiness or hopelessness, chronic feelings of 'being on edge' as if constantly threatened, and estrangement.

Alcohol and drug abuse may develop secondarily in torture survivors as a way of blocking out traumatic memories, regulating affect, and managing anxiety. Other possible diagnoses include: generalized anxiety disorder, panic disorder, acute stress disorder, somatoform disorders, bipolar disorder, delusional disorder, disorders due to a general medical condition (possibly in the form of brain impairment with result-ant fluctuations or deficits in level of consciousness, orientation, attention, concentra-tion, memory, and executive functioning), and phobias such as social phobia and agoraphobia.

COMPONENTS OF THE PSYCHOLOGICAL/ PSYCHIATRIC EVALUATION

The following is a list of the components of psychological/psychiatric evaluation of torture survivors:

Identifying data

- Patient's name, age, ethnicity, country of origin, marital status, and number of children.

- Referral source.

- Summary of collateral sources (such as medical, legal, and psychiatric records).

- Methods of assessment utilized (interviews, symptom inventories and check-lists, neuropsychological testing, etc.).

History of torture and ill-treatment

- History of torture.

- Persecution.

- Refugee displacement.

- Other relevant traumatic experiences.

Current psychological complaints

The assessment of current psychological functioning constitutes the core of the eval-uation. One should specifically inquire about the three DSM-IV categories of PTSD symptoms.

Post-torture history

This component of the psychological evaluation obtains information about current life circumstances and stresses.

Pre-torture history

- Developmental history.

- Family history: family background, family illnesses, family composition.

- Educational history.

- Occupational history.

- History of past trauma: childhood abuse, war trauma, domestic violence, etc.

- Cultural and religious background.

The summary of pre-trauma history is important to assess mental health status and level of psychosocial functioning of the torture victim prior to the traumatic events. In this way, the interviewer can compare the current mental health status with that of the individual before he or she was tortured. In evaluating background information the interviewer should keep in mind that the duration and severity of responses to trauma is affected by the severity and duration of the trauma events, genetic and biological pre-disposition, developmental phase, age, prior trauma, pre-existing personality, and social support system.[41]

Medical history

The medical history summarizes pre-trauma and current health conditions.

Past psychiatric history

One should enquire whether the individual has a past history of mental or psychological disturbances, the nature of the problems, and whether they received treatment or required psychiatric hospitalization. Enquire that if any psychotropic medications were used in treatment.

Substance use and abuse history

The clinician should enquire about substance use before and after the torture, changes in the pattern of use and abuse, and whether substances are being used to cope with insomnia or psychological/psychiatric problems.

Mental status examination

The mental status examination begins the moment the clinician meets the subject. The interviewer should make note of the person's appearance (such as signs of malnutrition, lack of cleanliness, etc.), changes in motor activity during the interview, use of language, presence of eye contact, and the ability to relate to the interviewer. The following list summarizes the components of the examination: general appearance, motor activity, speech, mood and affect, thought content, thought process, suicidal and homicidal ideation, and cognitive status (orientation, long-term memory, intermediate recall, and immediate recall).

Assessment of social function

Trauma and torture can affect a person's ability to function. The psychological consequences of the experience may impair the individual's ability to care for him/herself, earn a living, support a family, or pursue education. The clinician should assess the individual's current level of functioning by inquiring about daily activities, social role function (as housewife, student, worker, etc.), social and recreational activities, and perceptions of health status. For obvious reasons, one cannot accurately assess the social functioning of an individual held in detention.

Psychological testing and the use of checklists and questionnaires

If an individual has trouble expressing in words his or her experiences and symptoms; it may be useful to use a trauma event questionnaire or symptom checklist. These tools may facilitate disclosure of severely traumatic memories and reduce the anxiety often experienced in an unstructured interview. There are numerous questionnaires available; however, none is specific to torture victims. Caution must be exercised in the interpretation of responses and scores because established norms do not exist for most refugee populations. Similarly, there is little published information about the use of standard psychological and neuropsychological tests among torture survivors. Due to the fact that there is such wide cultural and linguistic diversity among this group, one should exercise extreme caution when requesting or employing psychological and psychometric tests of any kind, most of which have not been cross-culturally validated.

Clinical impression

Interpretation of the clinical findings is a complex task. The following questions from the Istanbul Protocol will help guide the formulation of the clinical impression and diagnostic conclusions.

1. Are the psychological findings consistent with the alleged report of torture?

2. Are the psychological findings expected or typical reactions to extreme stress within the cultural and social context of the individual?

3. Given the fluctuating course of trauma-related mental disorders over time, what is the timeframe in relation to the torture events? Where in the course of recovery is the individual?

4. What are the co-existing stresses impinging on the individual (e.g. ongoing persecution, forced migration, exile, loss of family and social role, etc.)? What impact do these issues have on the victim?

5. What physical conditions contribute to the clinical picture? Pay special attention to head injury sustained during torture and/or detention.

6. Does the clinical picture suggest a false allegation of torture?[6]

When writing reports, clinicians should comment on the emotional state of the person during the interview, symptoms, history of detention and torture, and personal history prior to torture. Factors such as the onset of specific symptoms in relation to the trauma, the specificity of any particular psychological findings, as well as patterns of psychological functioning should be noted. Additional factors such as forced migration, resettlement, difficulties of acculturation, language problems, loss of home, family, social status, as well as unemployment should be discussed. The relationship and consistency between events and symptoms should be evaluated and described. Physical conditions such as head trauma or brain injury may require further evaluation.

It is possible that some people may falsely allege torture or exaggerate a relatively minor experience or symptoms for personal or political reasons. The clinician should keep in mind, however, that such fabrication requires a detailed knowledge about trauma-related symptoms that individuals rarely possess. Also, inconsistencies can occur for a number of valid reasons such as memory impairment due to brain injury, confusion, dissociation, cultural differences in perception of time, or fragmentation and repression of traumatic memories. Additional sessions should be scheduled to help clarify inconsistencies and when possible, family or friends may be able to corroborate detail.

Recommendations

The recommendations depend on the original objective of the evaluation. The goal may be for legal matters such as asylum or resettlement, or for treatment. Recommendations can include further assessment such as neuropsychological testing, medical or psychiatric treatment, and/or need for security or asylum.

TREATMENT CONSIDERATIONS

A full discussion of treatment is beyond the scope of this chapter. To summarize, intervention necessarily begins with establishing safety, protection, and basic human necessities for survival (food, shelter, income, etc.). Without these basic elements, no meaningful 'treatment' can be effective. Any meaningful clinical treatment and rehabilitation programme should include social services and if possible, legal services. Treatment can begin once basic necessities are secured, or perhaps even while they are being secured. Because torture affects an individual at so many levels, an integrated, coordinated multi-disciplinary approach to treatment is essential. Mental health treatment modalities include individual, group, and family psychotherapy, psychopharmacology, psychoeducation, and somatic therapies. Traditional medicine practices should be respected and included in the treatment if the individual wishes, provided they are safe and that one avoids deleterious interactions between medications and herbal preparations.

REFERENCES

1   Keller AS, Eisenman DP, Saul J. Evaluating and treating the psychological consequences of torture. J Gen Intern Med 1997; 12(suppl 1):121
2   Goldfeld AE, Mollica RF, Pesavento BH, Faraone SV. The physical and psychological sequelae of torture: symptomatology and diagnosis. JAMA 1988; 259:2725–2729

3   Friedman M, Jaranson J. The applicability of the post-traumatic concept to refugees. In: Marsella T et al (eds), Amidst Peril and Pain: The Mental Health and Wellbeing of the World's Refugees. Washington, DC: American Psychological Association Press, 1994, pp 207–227

4   General Assembly Resolution 39/46, Annex, 39 UN. GAOR suppl (No. 51) at 197, UN Doc. A/39/51 (1984) entered into force 26 June 1987, Article 2

5   Declaration of Tokyo. Adopted by the World Medical Association in 1975

6   Istanbul Protocol (see: Welsh J. The problem of torture, Chapter 1 in this book)

7   Iacopino V. Treatment of survivors of political torture: commentary. J Ambul Care Manag 1998; 21(2):5–12

8   Somnier F, Vesti P, Kastrup M, Genefke IK. Psychosocial consequences of torture: current knowledge and evidences. In: Bosoglu M (ed.), Torture and its Consequences: Current Treatment Approaches. Cambridge: Cambridge University Press, 1992, pp 56–71

9   Allodi F. The psychiatric effects in children and families of victims of political persecution and torture. Dan Med Bull 1980; 27:229–232

10 Kleinman A. Anthropology and psychiatry: the role of culture in cross-cultural research on illness and care. Paper delivered at WPA 1986 Regional symposium on 'Psychiatry and its Related Disciplines'

11 Engelhardt HT. The concepts of health and disease. In: Englehardt HT, Spicker SF (eds), Evaluation and Explanation in the Biomedical Sciences. Holland: D. Reidel Publishing Co, 1975, pp 125–141

12 Westermeyer J. Psychiatric diagnosis across cultural boundaries. Am J Psych 1985; 142(7):798–805

13 Sartorius N. Cross-cultural research on depression. Psychopathology 1987; 19(2):6–11

14 Iacopino V, Allden K, Keller A. Health Professionals Guide to Assisting Asylum Seekers: Medical and Psychological Evaluation of Torture. Boston: Physicians for Human Rights (in press)

15 Wilson JP, Raphael B. International Handbook of Traumatic Stress Syndromes. New York: Plenum Press, 1993

16 Eisenbruch M. Commentary: Toward a culturally sensitive DSM: cultural bereavement in Cambodian refugees and the traditional healer as taxonomist. J Nerv Mental Dis 1992; 180:8–10

17 Weine SM et al. Psychiatric consequences of 'Ethnic Cleansing': Clinical assessments and trauma testimonies of newly resettled Bosnian refugees. Am J Psych 1995; 152:536–542

18 Schacter DL. Memory Distortion: How Minds, Brains, and Societies Reconstruct the Past. Cambridge, Massachusetts: Harvard University Press, 1994

19 Southwick SM, Morgan CA, Nicolaou A, Charney D. Consistency of memory for combat-related traumatic events in veterans of operation desert storm. Am J Psych 1997; 154:2, 173–177

20 Lopes Cardozo B, Vergara A, Agani F, Gotway C. Mental health, social functioning, and attitudes of Kosovar Albanians following the war in Kosovo. JAMA 2000; 284(5):569–577

21 Mollica RF, McInnes K, Pham T, Smith Fawzi et al. The does–effect relationships between torture and psychiatric symptoms in Vietnamese ex-political detainees and a comparison group. J Nerv Mental Dis 1998; 186(9):543–553

22 Wolfe J, Charney DS. Use of neuropsychological assessment in posttraumatic stress disorder. Psychol Assess J Consult Clin Psychol 1991; 3:573–580

23 Sutker P, Vasterling J, Brailey B, Allain A. Memory, attention, and executive deficits in POW survivors: contributing biological and psychological factors. Neuropsychology 1995; 9(1):118–125

24 Thygesen P, Hermann K, Willanger R. Concentration camp survivors in Denmark: persecution, disease, disability, compensation. Dan Med Bull 1970; 17:65–108

25 Eitinger L. Concentration Camp Survivors in Norway and Israel. London: Allen and Unwin,1964

26 Rasmussen OV. Medical aspects of torture. Dan Med Bull 1990; 37:1–88

27 Bostwick JM. Neuropsychiatry of depression. In: Ellison JM, Weinstein CS, Hodel-Malinofsky (eds), The Psychotherapist's Guide to Neuropsychiatry: Diagnostic and Treatment Issues. Washington, DC: American Psychiatric Press,1994, pp 409–431

28 Krystal J, Southwick S, Charney D. Posttraumatic stress disorder: psychological mechanisms of traumatic remembrance. In: Schacter DL (ed.), Memory Distortion. Cambridge, Massachusetts: Harvard University Press, 1995, pp 150–172

29 Krystal JH, Kosten TR, Perry BD Southwick S, Mason JW, Giller EL. Neurobiological aspects of PTSD: review of clinical and preclinical studies. Behav Therapeut 1989; 20:177–198

30 Sapolsky RM. Stress, the aging brain and the mechanisms of neuron death. Cambridge, Massachusetts: MIT Press, 1992

31 Freud S, Breuer J. On the psychological mechanism of hysterical phenomena. In: Jones E (ed.), Sigmund Freud, LLD Collected Papers, Vol. 1. London: Hogarth Press, pp 24–41

32 American Psychiatric Association. Diagnostic and Statistical Manual of Mental Disorders, 4th edn. Washington, DC: APA, 1994

33 Mollica RF, Donelan K, Tor S et al. The effect of trauma and confinement on the functional health and mental health status of Cambodians living in Thailand–Cambodia border camps. JAMA 1993; 270:581–586

34 Kinsie JD, Boehnlein JK, Leung P et al. The prevalence of posttraumatic stress disorder and its clinical significance among Southeast Asian refugees. Am J Psych 1990; 147(7):913–917

35 Allden K *et al.* Burmese political dissidents in Thailand: trauma; and survival among young adults in exile. Am J Public Health 1996; 86(1):561–569

36 Mollica RF, McInnes K, Sarajlic N, Lavelle J, Sarajilic, Massagli M. Disability associated with psychiatric comorbidity and health status in Bosnian refugees living in Croatia. JAMA 1999; 282(5):433–439

37 Marsella AJ, Friedman M, Spain H. A selective review of the literature on ethnocultural aspects of PTSD. PTSD Res Quarter 1992; 3:1–7

38 Remennick L. Stress and coping in the Israeli context: the role of cumulative adversity. Paper presented at the International Forum for Social Science and Health Regional Meeting. 21–23 April 2000 Istanbul, Turkey

39 Simpson MA. What went wrong? Diagnostic and ethical problems in dealing with the effects of torture and repression in South Africa. In: Kleber RJ, Figley CR, Gersons BPR (eds), Beyond Trauma – Cultural and Societal Dynamics. New York: Plenum Press, 1995, pp 188–210

40 World Health Organisation. The ICD-10 Classification of mental and behavioural disorders and diagnostic guidelines. Geneva, 1994

41 Van der Kolk BA. The psychological consequences of overwhelming life experiences. In: van der Kolk BA (ed.), Psychological Trauma. Washington, DC: American Psychiatric Press, 1987, pp 1–30

8

PHYSICAL EXAMINATION FOLLOWING ALLEGATIONS OF RECENT TORTURE

Onder Ozkalipci

INTRODUCTION

Getting a very detailed story will guide the physician who is searching for torture-related lesions on the body of the victim. This will include information about torture methods; a detailed account of the patient's physical and psychological complaints during and after the infliction of torture, and at the time of the examination; and the patient's observations of the acute lesions and the subsequent healing process. Acute lesions are often characteristic since they show a pattern of inflicted injury that differs from non-inflicted injuries, for example by their shape, repetitiveness, and distribution on the body.

After inspection of whole body, injured areas should be palpated so that tenderness and swelling can be determined. During the examination of skin injuries, location, size, and shape should be noted in detail for each lesion, together with the colour compared to surrounding skin (the same, lighter or darker), depth, swelling, oedema, crust, scab, ulceration, blistering, and any evidence of secondary skin infection.

After performing systematic evaluation of the cardiovascular, respiratory, and central nervous systems, special attention should be given to possible problems that may be suggested by the history of torture. For instance, in patients who report electric torture of the upper limbs, in addition to searching for traces of electrical burns, emphasis should also be put on examining for problems of the upper spine and the shoulder joint (tendon lesions, impingement, dislocation, and subluxation) that might have been caused by the muscle spasms.

The examiner should note all pertinent positive and negative findings using, where appropriate, body diagrams such as those in Appendix 3 of the Istanbul Protocol[1] to record the location and nature of all injuries. Then he or she should refer the patient for any necessary consultations and examinations, then call the patient back for a follow up examination. Some forms of torture such as electrical shock and blunt trauma may not have detectable findings initially, but they may be detected on subsequent examination. Photography should be a routine part of examinations.

Injuries that can be observed on the body include the following:

Abrasions

An abrasion is a scraping away of the superficial portions of the epidermis or destruction of the superficial layers by tangential application of force against the rough surface of the blunt object. Abrasions are more commonly observed over bony prominences or where a thin layer of skin overlies bone. When the blunt instrument scrapes off the superficial layers of the skin the surface is striped. If abrasions are deep and extend down to the dermis, capillaries may bleed, and serosanguineous fluid deposits on the surface of the skin that forms a brownish scab when it dries out.[2]

The abrasion remains moist until it forms a scab which consists of hardened exudate. The scab organizes in a few days and covers the lesions for up to a few weeks, then it usually leaves a pink intact surface after detaching. The pink colour gradually fades, reaching within a few months the final colour with respect to the surrounding skin.

Sometimes abrasions are linear, in which case they are called a scratch. These are caused by pointed objects such as wire-ends and pins. Sometimes victims of torture may be thrown from moving vehicles so that they slide on the road, or they may be dragged out on the ground during arrest or capture. In these cases extensive abrasions may be seen, and particles of dirt, sand, etc. will predispose the abrasion to infection.

Abrasions may show a pattern that reflects the contours of the instrument or surface that inflicted the injury. Elongated broad abrasions can be caused by the friction on the skin from objects such as ropes and cords. When the blunt force is directed perpendicular to the skin over the bony prominences, it will generally crush the skin at that point. Sometimes if there is anything between the object and the skin, its imprint may be observed on the skin. In hanging and other asphyxiations by ligature, patterned abrasions can often be found on the neck.

Contusions

A contusion or bruise is caused when blunt trauma occurs to the subcutaneous tissue resulting in rupture of blood vessels with extravasation into the neighbouring soft tissue. The continuity of the skin surface is unbroken. Contusions may be present not only in skin but also in muscles and internal organs.

The extent and severity of a contusion is related with the amount of force applied, but more importantly vascular structure of the traumatized area affects them. Elderly people and children who have loosely supported vascular structure will bruise more easily than young adults. Many medical conditions are associated with easy bruising or purpura, including blood disorders, vascular disorders, and vitamin and other nutritional deficiencies. Parts of the body with thin, lax skin and fatty areas bruise more easily.

Sometimes the shape of the bruise helps to identify shape of the blunt instrument that caused the injury. For example, rail-shaped bruising may occur when an instrument such as a truncheon or cane has been used.

Contusions that develop in the deeper subcutaneous tissues may not be observed for several days after injury, when the extravasated blood has reached the surface. Therefore, in cases when there is an allegation of blunt force but no sign of a contusion, re-examination after several days should be performed. It must be remembered that the final position and shape of such bruises bear no relation to the original trauma, and that other lesions may have faded by the time of re-examination.[3]

A haematoma is a focal collection of blood in the area of bruise.

Lacerations

Lacerations are a tearing or crushing of the skin and underlying soft tissues by the pressure of blunt force. They develop easily on the protruding parts of the body since the skin is compressed between the blunt object and the bone surface under the subdermal tissues. However, with sufficient force the skin can be torn on any portion of the body.

Incisions

Incisions are sharp trauma wounds that are produced when the skin is cut with a sharp object such as a knife, bayonet, or broken glass. Such wounds include cuts, stab wounds, and puncture wounds. The acute appearance is usually easy to distinguish from the irregular and torn appearance of lacerations.[4]

Burns

Burning is the form of torture that most frequently leaves permanent changes in the skin. Sometimes they may be of diagnostic value. Burns from torture are generally from contact with either hot materials or chemical substances. The level of the damage caused by application of hot objects depends on the intensity of heat and duration of exposure. First-degree burns are seen as reddening, but they have usually faded by the time the victim can consult a doctor. The classical appearance of second-degree burns is a moist, red, blistered lesion with complete destruction of the epidermis and partial destruction of basal layers. Sometimes third-degree burns are seen, with complete destruction of all layers of the skin. The shape of the lesions may or may not reflect the shape of object that caused the thermal injury.

Although it is more common for lit cigarettes to leave second- and third-degree burns, first-degree burns can be detected in rare cases. Cigarette burns often leave a circular or ovoid moist reddening, 5–10 mm in diameter, with subepidermal oedema and blister formation. A careful examiner may sometimes observe burnt hairs around the lesion. The cigarette fire has a conical structure and its intensity may change on different parts of the surface. Sometimes there is indistinct blister formation and the lesion is deeper in one part, with blisters partially or totally surrounding it. There may be complete disruption of the epidermis and most of the basal layer. In the later phase yellowish-green purulent exudate or ulcerative lesions may be observed in the base of the lesion. A thick crust forms, then the yellowish-green colour may be observed on the brown crust (Figure 8.1).[5]

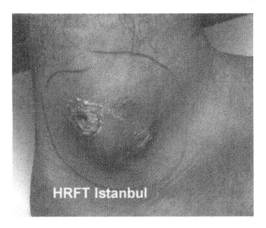

Figure 8.1 – Thirty-six hours after cigarette burn

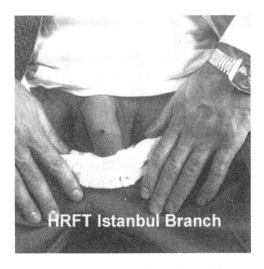

Figure 8.2 – Five days after an electrical burn

Trace electrical burns are usually a red-brown circular lesion, 1–3 mm in diameter, usually without inflammation, which may result in a hyperpigmented scar. The skin surfaces involved must be examined carefully because the lesions are often not easily discernible. Electrical burns may produce specific histologic changes,[6] but these are not always present, and the absence of such changes in no way mitigates against the lesion being an electrical burn. The decision must be made on a case-by-case basis as to whether or not the pain and discomfort associated with a skin biopsy can be justified by the potential results of the procedure (Figures 8.2 and 8.3).

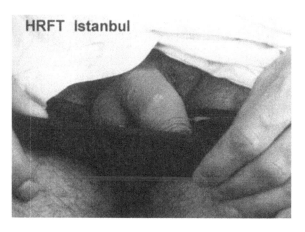

Figure 8.3 – The same lesion, 14 days after the electrical burn

Bite marks

The human bite is ovoid or elliptical in pattern and more blunt in appearance than those of under mentioned animals. Petechiae caused by sucking are only seen in human bite marks. These marks can easily be seen 1–24 h after infliction, and the assault from which they originate is generally sexual in nature.

Animal bites are characterized by puncturing and tearing of tissues, whereas the human bite compresses. Dog bites have a narrow squarish arch anteriorly, and the prominent pointed marks are produced by the canines. Cat bites have a small rounded arch, their puncture marks are also made by canines. The bites are often associated with scratch mark from claws. Rodents leave small bites caused by central incisors.[7]

Aging

Speculative judgments should be avoided in the evaluation of the nature and age of blunt traumatic lesions since a lesion may vary according to the age, sex, condition, and health of the patient, the tissue characteristics, and the severity of the trauma. Fresh and old injuries can be seen together on people who have a long history of torture.

Irradiation, corticosteroids, scurvy, diabetes, hepatic cirrhosis, uraemia, denervation of the wounded area, blood loss, cold, concussion, and shock all inhibit wound healing.[8,9] Wounds heal faster in young people. Bruises resolve over a variable period, ranging from days to weeks. Reddish-blue, blue or purplish-black bruises are almost certainly recent. As the extravasated red cells are destroyed, the aging bruise goes through variable colour changes of bluish-green, greenish-yellow and brown.

Estimating the age of non-recent bruises is one of the most contentious areas of forensic medicine.[10]

Fractures

Fractures are caused by a loss of bone integrity due to the effect of a blunt mechanical force on various vector planes. A direct fracture occurs at the site of impact or at the site where the force was applied. In an indirect fracture, the location, contours, and other characteristics of a fracture reflect the nature and direction of the applied force. The most frequent fractures seen in survivors of torture are of the nasal bones, the ribs, the radius, ulna and small bones of the hand, the transverse process of vertebrae, and those of the coccyx. The hyoid bone and laryngeal cartilage may be fractured in partial strangulation or from blows to the neck.

Routine radiographs are recommended at the initial examination, if facilities are available. Injuries to tendons, ligaments, and muscles are best evaluated with MRI, but arthrography can also be performed. In the acute stage, MRI can detect haemorrhage and possible muscle tears. Muscles usually heal completely without scarring, so later imaging studies will be negative. MRI or scintigraphy may detect bone injury such as a subperiosteal haematoma, which may not be detected on routine radiographs or CT.[11] Radiographic aging of relatively recent fractures should be done by an experienced trauma radiologist.

PHYSICAL EXAMINATION OF MUSCULOSKELETAL SYSTEM

Complaints of musculoskeletal aches and pains are very common in survivors of torture.[12] They may be the result of repeated beatings, of suspension, or of other positional torture. They may also be somatic. They are non-specific, but should be documented. In accordance with the characteristics of torture, complaints are characterized as pain in the respective region of the body, limitation of joint movement, swelling, paraesthesiae, numbness, loss of sensation to touch, and tendon reflex loss.

Physical examination of the skeleton should include testing for mobility of joints, the spine and the extremities. Pain with motion, contractures, strength, evidence of compartment syndrome, fractures with or without deformity, and dislocations should all be noted after documenting visible signs such as contusions, abrasions, and lacerations as described above. Trauma to muscle should be checked for, such as muscle rupture and muscle tearing. Specific clinical signs of ligament tear include swelling, bruising, muscle spasm, and painful stress test, often with joint laxity. There may be a palpable gap in the ligament. If it is completely torn, then considerable swelling and bruising occurs. Tendon ruptures, avulsions from the insertion of the bone, and dislocation of a tendon from its groove may all be observed.

NEUROLOGICAL EXAMINATION

The neurological examination should evaluate the cranial nerves, sensory organs and peripheral nervous system, checking for both motor and sensory neuropathies related to possible trauma. Performing examination of reflexes is important. Radiculopathies, other neuropathies, cranial nerve deficits, hyperalgesia, paraesthesiae, hyperaesthesia, change in position and temperature sensation, motor function, gait and coordination may all result from trauma associated with torture. In patients with a history of dizziness and vomiting, vestibular examination should be conducted, and evidence of nystagmus noted.

Head trauma

Head trauma is among the most common forms of torture. Repeated head trauma, even if not always of serious dimensions, can lead to cortical atrophy, and diffuse axonal damage. Scalp bruises are frequently not visible externally unless there is swelling. Bruises also may be difficult to see in dark skinned individuals, but will be tender to palpation.

Having suffered blows to the head, the torture survivor may complain of continuous headaches. These are often somatic, or may be referred from the neck. He or she may claim that there is pain when touched in that region, and diffuse or local fullness or increased firmness may be noted on palpation of the scalp. Headache may also be the initial symptom of an expanding subdural haematoma. There may be associated psychological changes of acute onset, and a CT scan or MRI must be arranged urgently, if one is available. It may also be appropriate to arrange psychological or neuropsychological assessment.

Soft tissue swelling and/or haemorrhage will usually be detected with CT or MRI. In cases of trauma caused by falls, contracoup lesions of the brain may be observed on investigation (on the opposite side to the point of impact), whereas following direct trauma, the main damage to the brain may be seen directly under the point of impact.

Victims of violent shaking complain of recurrent headaches, disorientation, and mental status changes. This form of torture may produce cerebral injury without leaving any external marks, although bruises may be present on the upper chest or shoulders where the victim or his or her clothing has been grabbed. At its most extreme, cerebral oedema, subdural haematoma and retinal haemorrhage can be observed, and death has been reported.[13]

Eyes

Conjunctival haemorrhage, lens dislocation, subhyeloid haemorrhage, retrobulbar haemorrhage, retinal haemorrhage, and visual field loss may all be observed following torture. Referral to an ophthalmologist is recommended whenever there is a suspicion of ocular trauma or disease.

Ears

Blunt trauma to the external ear may result in haematoma. Cartilage necrosis and infection are likely sequelae if the ear is left untreated. Lacerations of the pinna vary from those of minor significance to complete amputation. Rupture of the tympanic membrane is a frequent consequence of harsh beatings. Prompt examination is necessary to detect tympanic membrane ruptures less than 2 mm in diameter, as they can heal within 10 days. Also Kristensen[14] has found that in 760 cases of traumatic tympanic membrane perforations diagnosed within 14 days of injury, 78.7% healed spontaneously.

The short- and long-term sequelae of significant injury to the middle and inner ear are hearing loss, vertigo, tinnitus, unsteadiness and, less commonly, facial nerve paralysis. An audiogram should be performed to assess injury to the ossicles and inner ear. A conductive hearing loss is usually due to a tear in the tympanic membrane and blood in the middle ear. A hearing loss of less than 40 dB suggests an ossicular chain dislocation. Sensorineural loss indicates cochlear or retrocochlear damage.[15]

Fluid may be observed in the middle and/or external ear. If otorrhea is confirmed by laboratory analysis to be CSF, then MRI or CT should be performed, if possible, to determine the fracture site. The radiographic examination of fractures of the temporal bone or disruption of the ossicular chain is best determined by CT, then hypocycloidal tomography, and lastly linear tomography.

Nose

The nose should be evaluated for alignment, crepitation, and deviation of the nasal septum. Initially soft tissue swelling may make interpretation difficult and it may be necessary to re-examine the nose after 48 h when this has subsided. Frequently there is an associated deviation of nasal septum which may result in nasal obstruction. For simple nasal fractures, standard nasal radiographs should be sufficient. Sometimes the fracture of the nasal bone includes the frontal process of the maxilla, and sometimes it extends to include ethmoid labyrinth. For complex nasal fractures and when the cartilaginous septum is displaced, and when rhinorrhea is present, CT and/or MRI are recommended.

Jaw, oropharynx and teeth

The oral cavity must be carefully examined. During the application of electric current to the mouth, the tongue, gingiva or lips may be bitten. Lesions might also be produced by forcing objects or materials into the mouth. Temporomandibular joint syndrome can be caused by electric current and blows to the face. It will produce pain in the temporomandibular joint, limitation of jaw movement, and in some cases subluxation of this joint.

A careful dental history should be taken and, if dental records exist, these should be requested. The patient should be referred to a dentist if there is any damage to the teeth. Mandibular fractures, avulsions or fractures of the teeth, broken prostheses, swelling of the gums, bleeding, pain, or loss of fillings from teeth can all result from direct trauma or electric shock torture. Dental caries and gingivitis should also be noted. Poor quality dentition may be due to conditions in detention, or may have preceded it. X-rays and MRI are suggested for determining the extent of soft tissue, mandibular and dental trauma.

Chest and abdomen

Examination of the trunk, in addition to noting lesions of the skin, should be directed toward detecting regions of pain, tenderness or discomfort that would reflect underlying injuries of the musculature, ribs or abdominal organs. The examiner must consider the possibility of intramuscular, retroperitoneal and intra-abdominal haematomas, as well as laceration or rupture of an internal organ. Ultrasonography, CT scans and bone scintigraphy should be used, when realistically available, to confirm such injuries.[16] Routine examination of the cardiovascular system, lungs and abdomen should be performed in the usual manner. Pre-existing respiratory disorders are likely to be aggravated in custody, and new ones may develop. Near asphyxiation often leaves no marks and may cause acute and chronic respiratory problems as well as other complications.

Rib fractures are a frequent consequence of beatings to the chest. If displaced, they may be associated with lacerations of the lung and possible pneumothorax. Fractures of the vertebral pedicles may result from direct blunt force. Fractures of lower right rib carry a 10% risk of hepatic injury.[17]

Following acute abdominal trauma, the physical examination must seek evidence of damage to abdominal organs or the urinary tract, but this examination is often negative. Gross haematuria is the most significant indication of kidney contusion. Organ injury may present on investigation as free air, extraluminal fluid, and areas of low attenuation, which may represent oedema, contusion, haemorrhage or a laceration. Peripancreatic oedema is one of the signs of acute traumatic and non-traumatic pancreatitis. Ultrasound is particularly useful in detecting subcapsular haematomas of the spleen. Peritoneal lavage may detect occult abdominal haemorrhage, but free abdominal fluid detected subsequently on CT scan might be from the lavage or haemorrhage; thus invalidating the finding. Renal failure due to crush syndrome may be seen acutely following severe beatings.[18]

Assessment for referral

The clinician should not hesitate to seek any further consultation and examination that he or she considers necessary for the evaluation. Those who need further medical and/or psychological care should be referred to appropriate services. During ongoing care, further evidence may be detected that may not have been foreseen. If there is a rehabilitation centre for torture survivors in the region, the clinician should contact them for further support and advice.

In countries where there is a tradition of systematic torture, and pressure on health care professionals, the examining clinician may also prefer to refer patients to specialists to increase the number of medical witnesses to the torture (e.g. consulting with a dermatologist for a simple contusion).

DIFFERENTIATION OF SELF-INFLICTED AND ACCIDENTAL INJURIES FROM TORTURE

It is extremely difficult to determine whether an injury is self-inflicted or accidental by evaluating only the distribution and shapes of traumatic lesions on the patient's body. A complete examination of torture must be made. A very detailed account should be taken, including torture methods applied, the patient's observations of acute lesions and the subsequent healing process, and physical and psychological complaints. A thorough physical and psychological examination should be performed with, if possible, any necessary investigations. An assessment should then be made of all the findings and their consistency with the history of torture. There should be a consistency between alleged history of torture and the known tradition in that particular region, so the examining physician must be aware of the torture practices in the region of origin of his or her patient.

If there are witnesses of the detention among the friends and relatives of the patient, they should also be interviewed. It is necessary to offer psychological support to the witnesses, because of the psychological trauma that they could have experienced. In the case of torture allegations, psychiatric interviews should be encouraged and facilitated. Whenever possible, several specialists should be involved in such a case and they should share their doubts about the case.

Some detainees incise themselves with sharp instruments to stop interrogation and torture, and go to a safer place such as a hospital. Generally these lesions are superficial skin incisions with no serious vessel or tendon trauma. The victims are open that they inflicted the wounds themselves. There must be a secondary gain for self-inflicted lesions.

Several studies have been conducted in the field of forensic psychiatry to assess the credibility of statements of victims of violence, for example, the medical reporting criteria aiming to assess the reliability of statements of victims alleging sexual violence.[20,21] These could be helpful in evaluating the consistency of the report of the person alleging torture.

Case 1

Allegations:

- male applied for medical report

- 45-year-old Turkish citizen, married with two children

- expelled from a European country seven months before, leaving his family behind

- detained at the Turkish airport and was accused of treason

- history of being interrogated at the airport police station, then blindfolded and sent to a detention centre for six months in atypical conditions

- he alleged being exposed to beatings and falanga (on average two sessions a day) every day during the first six weeks

- then arbitrary beatings and falanga twice a month, and several other torture methods

- released a month before application

- the day before the application, he was again attacked by three or four unknown people (allegedly police officers)

- he was accused of treason and again heavily beaten, but he was not detained this time

- at no time did he see any faces during the six-month period of detention or during the attack on the street

Medical findings:

- several abrasions in different parts of the body, mainly in left side, the majority being superficial and similar to each other

- the bruises were smaller than 3 cm on face and shoulders

- no physical findings consistent with falanga[19]

- no bone scintigraphy findings consisted with falanga[11]

- minimal psychological complaint, refused evaluation by a psychiatrist

Issues:

- he has an important benefit from a positive report

- six months of official interrogation has not been reported by any torture survivor in Turkey in the past 15 years

- the expulsion date was confirmed, but his family in Europe did not apply to any human rights organization during the six-month period

- there was no similarity between the known detention centres and defined detention centres

- the abrasions were similar in pattern to each other with the majority on the left side, which would be unusual following the type of assault he described

- some positive scintigraphy findings would be expected in a 45-year-old male subjected to long-lasting severe falanga up to one month before

Outcome:

- the patient was confronted with the contradictions and he agreed that his allegations were false

Box 8.1

Case 2

Summary of the case:

- male applied for a medical report

- 40-year-old Turkish citizen

- detained at the exit of Istanbul Airport

- claimed to have been detained and tortured

- inconsistent history

- several positive traumatic findings on the body, some consistent with burns

- psychiatrist decided to apply MMPI to the applicant

- clinical psychologist who evaluated the results of MMPI and had no information about the story of applicant decided he may have acute psychotic disorder or he is a malingerer

- secondary gain was to obtain a medical report which can facilitate his immigration to a developed country

- the patient was confronted with the contradictions and he agreed that his allegations were false

Box 8.2

When the claim is suspected to be false, it may be appropriate to seek a psychiatric opinion. Psychiatrists may wish to administer tests including Minnesota Multiphasic Personality Inventory (MMPI), Harvard Trauma Questionnaire, Hopkins Checklist, and Horowitz Impact of the Event Scale.

Although it is important to differentiate false torture allegations from real ones, it must be kept in mind that false torture claims are rarely made in countries where torture is widespread or systematic. For example, over 1800 people applied to the Istanbul Office of the Human Rights Foundation of Turkey between 1991 and September 2000, claiming to have been tortured. Of these, only three cases have been diagnosed as having been false torture claims with self-inflicted injuries.

It might be reasonable to assume that the majority of the self-inflicted lesions can be superficial and located in the easily reachable parts of the body. However, it is still impossible to draw such a general rule given the limited number of such cases.

Torturers and their lawyers employed by the state authorities often claim that all the traumatic lesions on the body of torture survivor are self-inflicted or inflicted by other detainees. This is a question that should be answered by the investigators and physicians who examine the applicant.

State authorities have to secure the conditions stated in international standards for detention and to apply UN Principles on the effective investigation and documentation of torture and other cruel inhuman or degrading treatment or punishment.[1] It is the quickest and cheapest way to diminish torture claims.

REFERENCES

1 Istanbul Protocol. See: Welsh J. The problem of torture, Chapter 1 in this book
2 Di Maio DJ, Di Maio VJM. Forensic Pathology. New York: Elsevier, 1989, p 87
3 Gürpinar S, Korur Fincanci S. Insan Haklari Ihlalleri ve Hekim Sorumlulugu (Human rights violations and responsibility of the physician). In: Birinci Basamak Için Adli Tip El Kitabi (Handbook of Forensic Medicine for General Practitioners). Ankara: Turkish Medical Association, 1999
4 Crane J. Injury. In: McLay WDS (ed.), Clinical Forensic Medicine. London: Greenwich Medical Media, 1996, pp 143–162
5 Bicer U et al. Bir Iskence Yontemi Sigara Sondurme-Olgu Sunumu, III. Adli Bilimler Sempozyumu. Kusadasi-Turkey: Nisan, 1998, pp 14–17
6 See: Danielsen L. The examination and investigation of electric shock injuries, Chapter 13 in this book
7 Clark D. Forensic odontology. In: McLay WDS (ed.), Clinical Forensic Medicine. London: Greenwich Medical Media, 1996, pp 287–296
8 Berg S. Die Altersbestimmung von Hautverletzungen. Z Rechtsmed 1972; 70:121

9   Gilsa B. Die Altersbestimmung von Hautwunden, Medical Dissertation, Würzburg 1976
10 Robinson SP. Principles of Forensic Medicine. London: Greenwich Medical Media, 1996
11 Lök V, Tunca M, Kapkin E *et al.* Bone scintigraphy as an evidence of previous torture. In: Human Rights Foundation of Turkey. Treatment and Rehabilitation Center Report. Ankara: HRFT, 1994, pp 91–96
12 Rasmussen OV. Medical aspects of torture. Dan Med Bull 1990; 37(suppl 1):1–88
13 Pounder D. Shaken adult syndrome. Am J Forensic Med Pathol 1997; 18:321–324
14 Kristensen S. Spontaneous healing of traumatic membrane perforations in man: a century of experience. J Laryngol Otol 1992; 106:1037–1050
15 Curran AJ, Timon CVI. Head and neck injuries. In: Jones BJ (ed.), Medico Legal Reporting in Surgery. New York: Churchill Livingstone, 1997, pp 106–126
16 See: Lök V, Aytaclar S. Radiodiagnostic approaches in the documentation of torture, Chapter 14 in this book
17 Feliciano DV, Patcher HL. Hepatic trauma revisited. Current Prob Surg 1989; 26:459
18 Malik GH *et al.* Acute renal failure following physical torture. Nephron 1993; 63:434–437
19 Bojsen-Moller F, Flagstad KE. Plantar aponeurosis and plantar architecture of the ball of the foot. J Anat 1976; 121:599–611
20 Einführung in die Aussagepyschologie und in die Praxis der Glaubwürdigkeitsbegutachtung von Opfern sexueller Gewalt im Auftrag von Strafgerichten in der BRD, Dipl. Psychologin Marion Anthoff Texte zum internatiolen Seminar in Istanbul: Staatlich verübte sexuelle Gewalt an Frauen, 1999, pp 34–42
21 Tully B. Statement validation. In: Canter D, Alison L (eds), Interviewing and Deception. Aldershot: Ashgate Publishing, 1999, pp 83–103

9

PHYSICAL EXAMINATION FOR LATE SIGNS OF TORTURE

Robert Kirschner, Michael Peel

INTRODUCTION

Often when a physician is asked to examine a patient for evidence of torture, it will be many months or years since the alleged incident or incidents. In this situation it is rare to be able to state categorically that the patient has been tortured, although careful history taking and examination can allow an experienced physician to support strongly the allegations of torture. However, it is rarely, if ever, possible to say confidently that a patient has not been tortured. The issue is the degree of consistency between the history and the physical signs. Thus it is almost impossible to give a strong opinion on whether or not an individual has been tortured without a reliable history. Even where there is a detailed history from other sources, the physician should still check those aspects relevant to the torture, and to gain more information about exactly what is alleged to have happened. This allows the physician to gain an impression of the accuracy of the patient's memory for the events, and to help him or her to identify those parts of the examination on which to focus. If the patient is too distressed to relate a history, the report on the physical examination should be secondary to a detailed psychological or psychiatric report.

Prior to completing the report, an attempt should be made to obtain the patient's prior medical records, both pre- and post-torture, to the extent that these might be available. The results of an examination for the late signs of torture can be more definitive if this information is available to the examining physician.

For each lesion, the physician must ask him- or herself whether it could be congenital, a consequence of an illness or a degenerative process, or the result of trauma. If the latter, is it more likely that it was caused accidentally, self-inflicted, or inflicted deliberately in the way the patient describes? In the report, the following terms are commonly used:[1]

- *Consistent:* a non-specific lesion that could have many causes, including that described by the patient, e.g. scarring of the knees

- *Highly consistent:* a lesion which could well have been caused in the manner described by the patient, but where there are a few other possible causes, e.g. incision scars from bayonets

- *Typical of:* the appearance of the lesion is that usually found in this type of torture, but there are some other causes, e.g. cigarette burns

Occasionally lesions will be found that can only have been caused in the way described by the patient. These should be described as being 'diagnostic of' the torture alleged, with an explanation of why other causes are extremely unlikely.

Sometimes the physician will find a lesion that could not have been caused in the way the patient describes. That is to say they are 'not consistent' with the allegation. This should not necessarily lead the doctor immediately to the conclusion that the patient is fabricating his or her story. There are many reasons why a victim of torture might mis-attribute a lesion. He or she might have been blindfolded when the lesion was caused, and the attribution was an assumption.[2] Some victims of torture assume that they had no scars on their body before the torture, and so will attribute a scar that was caused in childhood to the torture. If there is a plausible reason for the mistake, then this should be explained in the report. Otherwise the doctor needs to discuss the matter with the person who requested the examination.

At the end of the report, the physician will come to a final conclusion in similar terms as to his or her opinion on the consistency between the history of ill-treatment and the overall pattern of physical findings.

GENERAL EXAMINATION

The physician should start the examination by making a general assessment of the patient including the objective psychological state and demeanor. For example, how does the patient stand, walk, climb stairs, and sit down? Is the he or she agitated, subdued, or calm? It is important not to interpret calmness as not having suffered, as many victims of torture remain calm when describing their experiences. Is he or she well-presented, clean and tidy? If not, could the cause be poverty and lack of access to facilities, his or her cultural norms, or could this be a sign of depression? Does the patient look about right for his or her age, too young, or too old? In many places there has only been accurate recording of births for 20 years or less, and an older person giving a clearly inaccurate age might simply not know how old he or she is. Does the person look over- or under-weight? Are there signs that the weight has changed recently?

The usual pattern for examining the body is the head and neck first, then the upper limbs, then the chest, abdomen and back, then the lower limbs, and finally the buttocks and genital region. It does not matter if the doctor used a different order providing everything is examined. It is not usually necessary to make the patient disrobe fully for examination, as this can make many victims of torture feel agitated and exposed. The head and neck can be examined with the patient fully clothed. Then he or she can remove the shirt for the arms and upper body to be examined. A woman can leave her breasts covered except when they are examined. Then the patient can put on a T-shirt or gown and take off his or her other clothes except the underwear so that the abdomen and legs can be examined. Finally, if necessary, the underwear is removed for the buttocks and genitals to be examined. Watching the patient undressing and dressing provides useful information about the mobility of the upper and lower limbs, and any associated disability. However, the patient's modesty must be respected. A chaperone must always be offered when examining a patient if the physician is not of the same sex.[3]

Examination of the skin

It is essential to examine all skin surfaces of a patient alleging that he or she has been tortured, even where the allegations are of assaults limited to particular parts of the body. Only to examine those lesions indicated by the patient means missing potentially important information. There may be scars of which the patient was unaware, for example on the back. There may be scars relating to an incident that the patient had forgotten, for example running into barbed wire when escaping. Sometimes it can be helpful to be sure that there were no scars on a particular part of the body, for example, if the patient claims to have been assaulted again after the examination.

All scars should be documented, including those that the patient is clear were caused in incidents other than torture. The attribution of scars to causes other than torture will support a patient's credibility, but it is important not to read too much into this as some patients will be aware of this and use it, for example in a false allegation of torture to support an asylum claim.

All scars should be measured and described, with the detail of the description depending on the significance of the scar or scars to the final opinion. The significance may depend on the specificity of the scar for a particular instrument of injury, the location of the scar, and its relationship to other, similar scars. Scars that are less specific, but 'consistent' with the history could be described as follows:

'There are four scars, between 1.5 and 3 cm in diameter, on the right knee.'

Scars that are more specific, and 'highly consistent' with the history should be described in more detail:

'There is a bi-convex scar, 6 cm long and 1.5 cm wide at the widest, on the left flank, 8 cm above the left iliac crest.'

Generally scars should be described to the nearest 0.5 cm. Those under 5 mm should only be included if they are significant to the allegation.

Accurate drawings of individual scars can be helpful if they are executed competently, but poor drawings by unskilled artists can be counter-productive. Where possible, photographs should be taken of significant lesions. Ideally professional medical photographers should be used, but high quality photographs can be obtained with any 35 mm camera fitted with a macro lens. The newer, high-resolution digital cameras also produce excellent photographs. If the appropriate equipment is not available, it is better to take any photograph with a simple camera at the time the patient is seen, and to get further professional shots later if possible. It is good practice to take a photograph from which the patient can be identified before photographing individual lesions and, if the camera permits, for the date and time to be on the photograph. There must always be an indication of scale on close-ups. Flash on the camera can have the effect of 'flattening' the scar on the photograph so, if possible, it is good to repeat some photographs in sunlit conditions with the flash off.

Skin can be damaged by trauma in one of four ways. It can be bruised, it can be abraded, it can be torn, and it can be cut.[4] Bruises, or contusions, occur when superficial blood vessels rupture and there is haemorrhage into the tissues. In most cases this does not leave any sequelae, but in some skin types there can be residual hyperpigmentation from severe bruising for up to five or ten years after the incident. This hyperpigmentation reflects the location of the late bruising, so the pattern might not be significant, if there was tracking of blood after the original injury. Sometimes, for example after beating with whips of sticks, the hyperpigmentation is linear and can be quite characteristic.

Abrasions, or grazes, are where the surface of the skin has been rubbed off. As the dermis is not fully damaged, again there are rarely and lasting signs. However, deep or repeated abrasions can leave a pattern of hypo- or hyperpigmentation. One classical example of this is a circle of hyperpigmentation around the wrist, or more rarely the ankle, often with few hairs or hair follicles. This is the result of persistent or repeated application of tight ligatures or handcuffs.[5] Full thickness abrasions tend to leave large, irregular scars.

These areas of changed pigmentation must be differentiated from the late effects of skin diseases such as eczema, and vitamin deficiencies such as scurvy and pellagra. However, signs of vitamin deficiency might be an evidence of poor nutrition in detention, and lesions from recurrent skin infections, particularly of the lower limbs, could be the result of poor hygiene in detention.

Lacerations are caused by tearing of the skin and soft tissues as a consequence of blunt trauma. These can be caused, for example, by direct blows and by falls. The skin tears where it is tight, usually over bony surfaces, where there is little subcutaneous fat, and not necessarily where the trauma was directed. An understanding of the dynamics of the blow can help to assess whether or not the resulting scar is consistent with the alleged trauma. Incisions are cuts to the skin caused by sharp objects such as knives, bayonets, broken glass, and pieces of metal. Sometimes doctors use the term 'laceration' to describe an incision, but this is incorrect. When the wound is fresh there are ways to differentiate lacerations from incisional wounds, but once the wound has healed, the differences between the two types of scar are much less. Incisions tend to be linear or curved, and sometimes it is possible to identify the direction of the cut. Lacerations are more likely to be irregular. Some wounds can be part incision and part laceration. In general forensic practice, stab wounds are differentiated from other incisions because they are deeper than they are wide. When the wound has healed, this difference is less relevant.

Asymmetrical scars, those in unusual locations, and those with a diffuse spread of scarring all suggest a deliberate cause.[6] Some sharp objects leave a distinctive scar, such as the pointed military belt buckle still used by soldiers in the former Zaire. The clips sometimes used to give electric shocks can pull away in the consequent muscle spasm and can leave a small scar where the clip was applied. Signs of the wound having been sutured at the time of injury should be documented. Large incisions that have gaped leave large, bi-convex scars. Surgical scars must also be documented with, if possible, an idea of the nature of the operation and the skill of the surgeon. Some surgical scars could be the result of torture, for example that following the removal of a ruptured spleen. Relatively trivial wounds can leave large scars if they become infected, for example if the victim is kept in a flooded cell with no toilet facilities.

Linear depigmentation around the axillae, the abdomen, the back, and the thighs are more likely to be striae distensae, especially if there is associated laxity of the skin.[7] They are usually clustered and relatively symmetrical, and should not be mistaken for scars caused by whipping. However, striae themselves may be a consequence of rapid weight loss or gain, so will support an allegation of poor nutrition in detention.

Traditional healers, particularly in parts of Africa, make multiple parallel scars about 5 mm long over a painful part of the body.[2] They are relatively easy to differentiate as torture scars are rarely so small and neat. The other differential to bear in mind, particularly in patients of African origin, is tribal markings, especially on the face. Bullet wounds are usually distinctive, but are more likely to be caused by crossfire or during escape attempts than during torture.

Cigarette burns are typically round and a little less than 1 cm in diameter with a depigmented centre and a hyperpigmented periphery.[7] This appearance is unlikely to be caused by anything else, and the main differentials are that they were self-inflicted or, very rarely, inflicted by a friend to support a false claim of torture. Self-inflicted scars tend to be in accessible parts of the body, particularly inside the forearms and on the non-dominant side.[8] Those inflicted by friends are generally few and not particularly deep. Lighted cigarettes are one of the commonest tools of torturers, and there are a wide range of scars left by cigarettes that are less typical. Sometimes they are large end irregular, either from lit cigarettes being rubbed into the skin, or from many confluent burns. When the cigarettes are not pressed in firmly they can leave small areas of hyperpigmentation that fade after a few months or years. The individual scars might not be distinctive, but the number and distribution can be strongly supportive of a history of torture.

Burns from heated metal objects are generally sharply demarcated and atrophic, so have the shape of the part of the object touching the skin, but a little smaller because of the contraction of the scar. Scars from hot water or, less commonly, caustic substances, leave a pattern of scarring, depigmentation and hyperpigmentation in which the flow of liquid can be identified. Scars from melted plastic also show a flow, but they tend to be smaller as the plastic flows more slowly and cools more rapidly. A single scald could be from a domestic accident, but many scars on different parts of the body that could not have come from a single accident are very likely to be from torture. This is one of the situations when a detailed occupational history can be important. For example it could be suggested that a large burn scar on a man who has worked as a ship's officer could have been sustained when a boiler exploded. If it is known that the man was a deck officer who never needed to enter the engine room, this alternative hypothesis becomes much less tenable.

It must be stressed that a simple scar count is not the same as an expert opinion as to whether or not a patient has been tortured. Many victims of torture have no scars or other physical signs. A small number of distinctive scars can often be much more helpful than a large number of non-specific scars. Other possible causes of scarring must be considered and, where appropriate, documented. For example, it is difficult to support an allegation of being punched by the police in a man who was previously a professional boxer as there is no way to differentiate such scars. On the other hand, a number of victims of torture support themselves by working as casual labour on construction sites in an intermediate stage of their escape. Typical scars of construction workers are quite different from those commonly caused by torture. A large number of scars on a patient is more likely to be a sign of the impunity of the security services in the country of torture. Where there is even minimal judicial supervision the police and army are much more careful not to leave physical signs, and often keep the person incommunicado for several days before release to let the bruising fade.

Head and neck

The physical examination usually starts with the face. The patient may be particularly concerned about noticeable scars as they are a permanent reminder of the torture. Large rings on the hands of the assailant can leave quite distinctive scars, and if there are several people alleging torture by the same person, the similarity of the scars is important evidence. More commonly, scars on the face are quite small and need to be differentiated from those caused by childhood and adolescent trauma, infections such as acne and chickenpox, and tribal markings.

Victims who have spent many months in complete darkness often complain of a redness and soreness of the eyes in bright light for several years afterwards. The eyes can look red if the patient is seen on a sunny day, but there is no other abnormality visible. This phenomenon needs more investigation before it will be possible to reassure patients that it will go away.

Patients often complain that teeth have been knocked out, loosened, or damaged during assaults to the face. Fractures or chips of the upper incisors are particularly common. An assessment of dental trauma requires knowledge of the patient's pre-incarceration dental health. In those who previously had regular dental care, the presence of caries, periodontal disease or tooth trauma may be highly significant as a marker of prolonged detention and/or dental torture. However, where the patient's dental health was poor prior to detention, it is less likely that anything helpful can be said about allegations of dental trauma.

In a number of countries it is common to slap victims of torture around one or both ears with the palm of the hand, rupturing the eardrum ('telefono').[6] However, it is not unknown in many of those countries for teachers or parents to assault children in the same way. There are also allegations, particularly from the Indian sub-continent, of torturers pushing a pencil into the auditory canal then hitting it through the eardrum. Scars of the tympanic membrane from childhood ear infections tend to be symmetrical and circular, whereas those from trauma can be more stellate in shape. With experience, it can sometimes be said that a scar of the eardrum is likely to have been caused by torture, but never that the scar could not have been caused in this way. Audiometric tests can demonstrate hearing loss and support a history of relative deafness since the trauma.

Many victims of torture have been beaten repeatedly around the head and will have spent considerable periods unconscious or semi-conscious. Because of this, some parts of the history can be confused and illogical. There may be episodes that have been mis-remembered, and this must be allowed for in assessing the credibility of the patient. Permanent severe brain damage is relatively rare in survivors of torture, and its assessment should be left to an experienced neurologist or neuropsychologist. The examining physician should perform a routine neurological examination, including testing of the cranial nerves.

Many patients attribute headaches to their head injuries, but most survivors of torture complain of severe and repeated headaches and neck and back pain, irrespective of whether or not they had suffered loss of consciousness. Some patients with seizures say that they were caused by torture. This may be true, but it cannot be proven without good contemporaneous medical records.

X-rays of the skull may be helpful in documenting head trauma, and substantiating a claim of torture. Fractures of the orbit, nasal bones or zygoma sustained during torture may remain misaligned when they heal if medical care for the injury was denied.[9]

Chest and abdomen

Some victims of torture complain of persistent or recurrent chest pain. There are rarely any positive physical findings, although sometimes there is some costo-chondral tenderness. These patients can be reassured and, if possible, referred for physiotherapy. A chest X-ray can confirm the presence of healed rib fractures.

Victims of torture can be partially asphyxiated in a number of ways including having the head held under water that might be contaminated, having a plastic bag tied over the head, perhaps with a little petrol in it, forcing a cloth into the mouth and pouring fluid on it. Patients may give a history of recurrent infection or persistent cough, but usually these have settled by the time that patient is examined several months or years later. Sometimes patients say that they have been asthmatic since their torture, either following such partial asphyxiation of being forced to inhale smoke or tear gas.

The history in these cases is often convincing, but auscultation and measurement of flow rates rarely adds anything.

Stab wounds to the abdomen can be mistaken for surgical scars, especially if they have been sutured, but the history and the location of the scar are helpful in differentiating. Drain scars can be confused with scars unrelated to surgery, especially if they have not been sutured.

Back

It is important to inspect the back in detail, as many victims of torture are not aware of their scars. Once a scar is identified, the patient may remember an episode following which he or she was aware of bleeding. Others will say they have no idea how or when the scar was caused, and this should be documented. Whipping and beating with sticks can leave lines of hyperpigmentation as well as scarring.[2] Sometimes torturers embed small pieces of metal in whips, or hammer nails through sticks, and these can leave a distinctive appearance.

Most victims of torture complain of back pain, and the back is often tender to palpation. However, these findings are common in refugees who have not been tortured, and there are no distinctive physical signs.

Buttocks and genital region

Sometimes beatings of the lower back extend to the buttocks, and the linear scars and hyperpigmentation from whippings and beatings can be seen there. Most beatings of the buttocks and all assaults of the genitals are considered to be sexual torture, and are discussed in the sections on sexual torture of females and of males in Chapters 10 and 11 respectively.

Upper limbs

It is not normally necessary to check the pulse and blood pressure in the late documentation of torture, unless the data is needed for other purposes, but many doctors consider it good practice. It is important to bear in mind that the inside of the forearm is the commonest place for self-inflicted wounds. Those on the outside of the forearms could be from defence injuries, which would strengthen the support for an allegation of assault. Circles of hyperpigmentation around the wrist are likely to have been caused by handcuffs or other ligatures that were too tight or were rubbing. Vaccination scars should be identified and documented.

Victims of torture often claim that fingernails and toenails have been removed. Generally the nails grow back normally, and there is no way of telling that they have been removed. Even when the nails are mis-shapen, this is more likely to be the result of infection than permanent damage to the nail bed.

A palpable callus can be felt at fracture sites for many years, and may render X-rays unnecessary in some cases. Even with X-rays, it is rarely possible to state unequivocally that a fracture was caused by torture rather than in an accident, although healing with misalignment or fractures at unusual sites (e.g. transverse fractures through mid-radius and ulna) are highly supportive of a history of torture with no immediate medical treatment.

It is essential to conduct a neuromuscular examination of both upper and lower limbs to detect persistent musculoskeletal injury and/or motor or sensory nerve impairment. Examination of the shoulder following suspension is described in Chapter 10.

Lower limbs

The evaluation of scars on the legs is particularly difficult as many people who have not been tortured have scars there. However, scars from torture are more likely to be seen on the upper thighs and inside the thighs. Deep incisions of the thighs are likely to have been caused by torture, but burns of the front of the thighs could be accidental. Scars of the knees are almost invariably non-specific, and can *rarely* be said to be more than 'consistent' with allegations of torture. A small number of scars on the shins will be seen in many patients, especially if they played soccer or other contact sports in adolescence. Large numbers of scars on the legs are more likely to have been caused by torture. In patients from appropriate geographical regions, large irregular scars around the lower legs could have been caused by tropical ulcers in childhood.

Examination of the feet following allegations of falaka is described in Chapter 10.

REFERENCES

1   Istanbul Protocol. See: Welsh J. The problem of torture, Chapter 1 in this book
2   Forrest D. Guidelines for the Examination of Survivors of Torture, 2nd edn. London: Medical Foundation for the Care of Victims of Torture, 2000
3   See: Reyes H. Visits to prisoners and documentation of torture, Chapter 5 in this book
4   Crane J. Injury. In: McLay WDS (ed.), Clinical Forensic Medicine. London: Greenwich Medical Media, 1996, pp 59–73
5   Peel M, Hinshelwood G, Forrest D. The physiological and psychological findings following the late examination of victims of torture. Torture 2000; 10(1):12–15
6   Rasmussen OV. Medical aspects of torture. Dan Med Bull 1990; 37(suppl 1):1–88
7   Danielsen L. Skin changes after torture. Torture 1992; (suppl 1):27–28
8   Bunting R. Clinical examinations in the police context. In: McLay WDS (ed.), Clinical Forensic Medicine. London: Greenwich Medical Media, 1996, pp 59–73
9   See: Lök V, Aytaclar S. Radiodiagnostic approaches in the documentation of torture, Chapter 14 in this book

10

EXAMINATION FOLLOWING SPECIFIC FORMS OF TORTURE

Duncan Forrest

INTRODUCTION

Although physical torture as practised around the world has many features in common, almost invariably including beating, slapping and kicking, more sophisticated techniques have been developed in many areas.[1] In countries whose authorities wish to disguise the fact that torture takes place, methods are devised, sometimes with the help of doctors, that produce maximum pain with minimum external evidence. This must be recognised by the examiner if the after effects of these techniques are not to be missed, especially after the passage of time. Documentation of special methods of torture alleged by an individual requires that the examiner has a detailed knowledge of torture techniques used in the country where the torture was alleged to have taken place. With this knowledge the interviewer can take an informed and detailed history (taking care to avoid using leading questions). This helps to give a precise picture of such details of torture as the victim's posture, clothing, blindfolding or hooding, the implements used, duration of assault and his or her condition at the end of the session – whether he or she could walk or, whether there were any bleeding wound.[2,3] *It cannot be emphasised too strongly that such a detailed history is essential to ensure that during the subsequent physical examination signs in the relevant areas of the body are not missed and that a correct differentiation from accidental or self-inflicted injury is made.* For this reason the author makes no apology for describing at length some of the techniques employed in different countries before outlining the symptoms and signs to be expected during history taking and physical examination. Of particular value in assessing the severity of the attack is a history of loss of consciousness, though this should be elaborated by questions aimed at finding out whether unconsciousness was caused by blows to the head, asphyxiation, unbearable pain or exhaustion.

BEATING

When the aim is to disguise its effects, beating may be performed with heavy, flexible implements such as sandbags or lead-filled plastic pipes which may leave short-lived bruising but no permanent scarring. Sometimes the torturers perform the beating over clothing or folded towels. The impact of the blows is still severe and such beating may cause deep muscle bruising (which may take several days to reach the surface) or internal bleeding. This has been reported to lead to renal failure due to release of myoglobin.[4] In many countries severe beatings which cause widespread bruising is discontinued after the first few days of detention so that when the victim is produced to court or released after ten days or more, all signs of beating will have faded.

Falaka: It can be defined as the repeated beating of the feet. Although the term is occasionally used to describe beating on the hands, we will use the term in its narrow sense in this text and by this rather than by its alternative names of *falanga* or *bastinado*. The technique has been practised throughout history. It is still very common, not only in the Middle East, but also in the Indian subcontinent and, according to

Amnesty International, in over thirty countries worldwide. In some countries, such as Turkey, it is applied almost as a routine at the time of detention and many torture survivors report having suffered it on numerous occasions. It may be applied by batons, whips or canes to the barefeet or with shoes still on, and the immediate effect will depend on these variables. Often the victim is made to walk round on rough paving afterwards, sometimes carrying another on his back. This is clearly intended to add to the humiliation as well as the pain. The feet may be soaked in salt water afterwards, presumably to reduce swelling and for the same reason the shoes or boots are sometimes forced back on to the feet at the end of the session.

Early clinical state: The immediate effect is gross bruising and swelling and intense burning pain so that the diagnosis presents no difficulty. The victim will have obvious difficulty in standing and will be barely able to walk. Though not usual, there are sometimes open wounds on the soles. Examination will reveal marked tenderness and the feet must be handled very gently. Damage to toenails or fractures of the metatarsals or phalanges may be obvious for inspection and palpation but if not can be detected by X-ray or scintigraphy.[5,6]

Late results: Virtually all survivors of severe and repeated *falaka* complain of some symptoms for years afterwards though there is poor correlation between the extent of the history and the final severity of symptoms and signs. Typically, ability to walk long distances is limited, requiring a rest after every few hundred metres and, after much standing or walking during the day the pain increases at night when the warmth of the bed-clothes causes tingling or burning pain in the feet and calves and all the joints of the lower limbs. Sometimes relief is sought by walking on a cold floor or bathing the feet in cold water. The initial swelling may have resulted in deep destruction through ischaemia in the deep muscle compartments of the feet, so that at least some of the pain on walking may be caused by the so-called closed compartment syndrome[7,8] as first described in athletes. In cultures where squatting or sitting cross-legged are customary, the survivor may be greatly handicapped by his inability to take up these postures comfortably. On examination, the gait appears awkward, with loss of the normal easy rhythm and climbing stairs is clumsy. There may be roughness, scarring or pigmentation of the skin of the soles, significant in a subject who has habitually worn shoes but of doubtful significance in one who has spent a lifetime barefoot. The most constant sign is abnormal tenderness on deep palpation over the ball of the foot and plantar aponeurosis and pain on squeezing the heel. Roughness may be felt in the plantar aponeurosis. Movement of the toes often causes pain and ankle movement is limited by pain. If the cutaneous nerves have been traumatised, there may be either diminished sensation or paraesthesia in one or more toes and disruption of the autonomic pathways may cause sweating or hot or cold feet. In gross cases there is 'smashing of the heel' due to destruction of the fatty heel pads responsible for the normal shock-absorbing function so that when the heel strikes the ground on walking the impact is transmitted directly up the skeleton as far as the spine resulting in chronic aching pain in the shins, thighs, hips and back. A smashed heel becomes obvious on palpation – the bone can be felt directly under the skin of the heel – or on observing the flattened heel pads while viewing the standing subject from behind.[7] If there has been disruption of the plantar aponeurosis it is shown by an abnormal range of passive dorsiflexion of the great toes (more than 70 degrees).[7]

In most cases, though, the late signs are less florid, confined to marked localised tenderness and an abnormal pattern of walking which in themselves, while not diagnostic, give strong support to a history of *falaka*. *The diagnosis is not negated by the absence of gross signs.*

Special investigations: These include X-ray which occasionally reveals fractures or aseptic necrosis of one or more of the metatarsals.[9] Scintigraphy has been reported[5,6] as revealing areas of activity after *falaka* but we have not found it to be a reliable index after about six months. MRI scanning has been described as showing thickening of the plantar fascia.[10] So far there seems to be little more than could be discovered by manual palpation but more sophisticated techniques may in the future demonstrate deeper trauma such as pathology in the closed muscle compartments of the feet.

Treatment: Chronic state treatment includes gentle massage to the muscles of the feet, calves and thighs, re-education of the walking pattern and supportive footwear, especially designed to offer cushioning of the heels.

BLOWS TO THE EARS

Though punches and blows from batons or rifle butts may cause incidental damage to the ears, deliberately striking both ears simultaneously (*teléfono*) either with the flat of the hands, wet towels or flat implements is especially damaging. There may be immediate bleeding from one or both ears and deafness caused by rupture of the eardrum. There is often tinnitus for a while. Attacks of otitis media may supervene. Deafness usually gradually improves as the drum repairs itself. Small perforations can heal in about ten days. Very occasionally there is dislocation of the ossicles which will cause permanent loss of hearing. Even more rarely, a perilymph fistula my lead to vertigo. Few of the long-term signs are specific to torture, but a careful history may make the differentiation from disease possible and an expert may be able to differentiate a perforation resulting from trauma from one caused by infection.

TRAUMA TO THE EYE

Direct violence to the eye is very common, either incidental to general beating about the head or else intentionally aimed. There may be conjunctival or retinal haemorrhage, dislocation of the lens or detachment of the retina. Torturers often force their victims to look at the sun or bright lights for long periods. Conversely, detainees may be kept for months or years in total darkness. Survivors often complain long afterwards of lachrimation and photophobia. However, such cases do not show any detectable physical abnormality and treatment is purely symptomatic.

RESTRAINT, SHACKLING AND CRAMPED CONFINEMENT

Some degree of restraint is clearly necessary and legitimate at the time of arrest or during transfer in order to prevent a detainee from escaping. However, once detention has been secured, there can be no legitimate need for artificial restraint. The use of shackles or leg irons is specifically forbidden by Rule 33 of the UN Standard Minimum Rules for the treatment of prisoners. In spite of this ruling, extreme and prolonged measures are very often taken. Sometimes an attempt is made to justify their use as preventing escape but usually they are applied to cause humiliation or as a punishment. The restraint may be continued for days or even weeks, far longer than needed for legitimate purposes.

Handcuffs, wrist or ankle ties leave no mark if they are applied properly, and in some countries officers take care to prevent damage. In India, for instance, police often use the detainee's turban cloth to bind the wrists or ankles. Conversely, restraints may cause abrasions or bruising even after a short time if they are of rough or harsh material or are applied too tightly. Thin ligatures tightly applied may cause deep wounds after a few hours. The type of handcuff which automatically continues to tighten if the prisoner struggles, is particularly dangerous, and can cause characteristic lesions.

The use of *leg irons* is widespread in police stations and prisons. Pakistani prisons are particularly notorious for their use, often for long periods of time. They are used as punishment, as a means of extorting bribes and intimidating or humiliating prisoners. Often the rings round the ankles are roughly finished and cause severe abrasions and scarring which may be diagnostic.

The *'five-point tie'* is a technique of trussing up a captive used in several African countries. A single fine rope is tied round the wrists, ankles and neck or mouth, holding the trunk tightly in extreme extension. Every attempt to relieve the pain by moving one limb tightens it more round the others. If this type of restraint is continued for any length of time there is almost certain to be permanent scarring and perhaps peripheral nerve or vascular lesions.

In China, many forms of shackling are used as punishment and are given nicknames to disguise the appallingly painful methods used.[11] For instance, *Su Qin bei jian* (literally, 'Su Qin carries a sword on his back') describes the shackling of one arm pulled over the shoulder to the other which is twisted behind the back. Another is *liankao*, describing various methods of shackling the hands and feet behind the back.

Cramped or distorted postures or prolonged standing are used routinely in many countries. An example is Israel, where 'moderate physical pressure' is permitted by law. Several techniques have been devised by the General Security Service (*Shin Bet*) and routinely used to put detainees under undue stress.[1,12] In *shabeh* the victim is shackled for hours to a low chair whose front legs have been shortened so that he must constantly struggle to avoid sliding off. In *gambaz* the detainee is forced to crouch on his toes in the 'frog' position for long periods. In *kas'at tawila* the subject is made to kneel with his back up against a table and his cuffed arms resting on the table behind him while the interrogator's legs push against his shoulders. A small chamber nicknamed 'the refrigerator' is used to keep the victim immobile for hours or days.

SUSPENSION

This may be of several types. In the simplest, the victim is hung by the wrists tied in front of the trunk. There may be resultant scarring round the wrists but not usually any significant musculo-skeletal or neurological damage. More severe techniques of suspension are likely to cause additional temporary or permanent soft tissue injury to the limbs. Suspension by the arms or wrists tied behind the back is commonly known as '*Palestinian hanging*'. It is customary for the victim to be lifted off his feet for a few minutes at a time, perhaps beaten, given electric shocks or even have heavy weights tied to the legs, and then lowered for periods of recovery from the extreme pain. There is such an unnatural strain on all the muscles and ligaments of the shoulder girdle that one or both shoulders may dislocate. Victims complain for several days afterwards of inability to raise the arms above the head and sometimes of numbness and weakness of the fingers. For years afterwards they may experience pain on raising the arms, lifting weights or combing the hair. On examination there is usually tenderness in the muscles around the shoulders and scapulae and severe pain on passive movements, especially extension and internal rotation of the shoulders. There is occasionally winging of the scapulae caused by traction on the long thoracic nerve, easily missed unless specially looked for by asking the subject to press against a wall with outstretched arms, and there may be permanent deficit of the lower roots of the brachial plexus, as shown by sensory deficit in an ulnar distribution.

The *parrot's perch* (*pau de arara*, the chicken, the bar) is another form of suspension which causes immediate severe pain. It has been commonly used in many Latin American countries but is also seen in Africa. The wrists are bound together in front of the body, the arms passed over the knees and a pole thrust behind the knees. The result may be rupture of the cruciate ligaments or sensory or vascular damage below the knees.

There are many other methods of suspension including hanging by the ankles or with the arms tied to a cross-bar as in 'crucifixion'. Whether there will be any immediate or later ill-effects depends on the method used, the posture of restraint and the distribution of bonds which may have been not only at the wrists and ankles but also at any point of the arms, legs or trunk.

Suspension by the hair can avulse the scalp leading to an immediate cephalhaematoma which may persist and be palpable for months or even years as a boggy swelling.

In any event, the scalp is likely to remain tender, sometimes with the scalp attached unnaturally firmly to the underlying skull.

Examination: These methods of abuse may produce a variety of after effects, complicated by the fact that restraint or suspension is often accompanied by beating, so it is impossible to generalise, but if the examiner asks the subject to describe or mime the particular posture and stress he was subjected to, it is possible to decide what areas of skin, joints and muscle groups to concentrate on during physical examination. This entails a detailed search of the skin for marks of bonds, the joints for limitation of movement by pain or, occasionally, tendency to subluxation, and muscle groups for abnormal tension and tenderness as well as a neurological examination for peripheral nerve lesions and the extremities for vascular changes. Abnormalities are likely to be easily found in the immediate aftermath but usually fade with time. Unless the full thickness of skin has been destroyed by tight bonds there is unlikely to be any permanent scarring where bonds have been applied though they must be searched for. *Their absence does not negate the allegation.* In most cases all signs on the skin fade after a few days, but if abrasions become infected or there is deep destruction of skin, there will be permanent scarring, changes in pigmentation or occasionally, only depilation. Lesions are usually linear and transverse and most marked over bony prominences. These are suggestive, but only if they are almost completely circumferential round the limbs they are diagnostic of restraint and could not have been caused in any innocent way. Though usually situated at the level of the wrists or ankles, they may be found further up the limbs because bonds may be applied higher or ride higher up. In many cases joint movements remain limited and painful for months or years and tenderness of muscle groups is often persistent. Motor or sensory changes tend to improve with time.

Treatment: The sooner after injury that treatment can be instituted the better but it is rare for any professional care to be possible until long after the events. Victims often say that they were treated by traditional methods of massage and exercise, with relief of pain on their release from detention. Late treatment concentrates on physiotherapy with massage, graduated exercises and postural re-education. At first, the therapist must be extremely careful to respect the patient's fear of contact and may not even be able to touch him until a satisfactory rapport has been established.

CRUSHING AND STRETCHING INJURIES

Many torturers injure their victims by stamping on their hands or feet with heavy boots, leaving scarring and fractures of the digits, which may give a good indication of how the injuries were inflicted. However, it is not usually possible to differentiate nails damaged by trauma from the subjects of previous chronic infection.

'*Cheera*' is the Punjabi word for tearing. It is the nickname given to a technique common in the north-west of the Indian subcontinent.[13] The victim is seated on the floor, often with an officer behind him with a knee in his back and pulling the head back by the hair. The legs are stretched apart, either suddenly or gradually, until they reach as much as 180 degrees. There is often a sound and sensation of tearing and, of course, the pain is excruciating. Often there is the additional trauma of kicks aimed at the inner aspect of the thighs or the genitals. In extreme cases the femur may fracture. The usual immediate result is the appearance of extensive haematomata in the groins or lower on the inner aspect of the thighs depending on whether the adductors have been torn off their origins or the muscles of the bellies have been disrupted. Naturally, walking is almost impossible for a long time. The late findings are pain on walking long distances, tenderness over the origins or muscles of the bellies and extreme limitation of abduction of the hips by pain. If the legs have been kicked, there are sometimes circular or irregular scars on the inner aspect of the thighs, an unusual site for accidental trauma. On one occasion I have seen stretch marks in the skin of the groins, not a position one would expect naturally-occurring striae. It remains impossible to squat, kneel or sit cross-legged for months or years afterwards.

In the same part of the world the '*ghotna*' is routinely used in police stations and interrogation centres.[13] It is a traditional domestic implement, a pole about four feet long and four inches in diameter used for grinding corn or spices. In many police stations implements specially made of metal are used instead. These may be filled with concrete and extremely heavy. One was reported to have '75 kg' printed on it. The commonest method is, with the victim seated or lying supine on the floor, for the *ghotna* to be rolled up and down the front of the thighs with one or more of the heaviest policemen standing on it. Occasionally, with the victim prone, it is rolled over the buttocks and back of the thighs or calves, but it is usual for bony areas like the shins to be avoided. The immediate effects are extensive bruising and inability to walk and even years later there is usually pain on walking far. On examination there is always marked tenderness on squeezing the thigh muscles. Occasionally areas of fat necrosis can be palpated. If a rough or angular log has been used there may be some scarring of the skin. Sometimes scars are found over the anterior superior spine, the patellae or the shins.

Another way for the *ghotna* to be used is, with the victim lying prone, the *ghotna* to be placed behind the knees and then the legs bent forcibly over it, straining and possibly disrupting the cruciate ligaments. The late effects of this depend on the amount of internal damage to the knee joints that has been caused. If severe, there may be permanent difficulty in walking, tenderness on palpating the joint margins and marked limitation by pain of flexion of the knees. Squatting, kneeling or sitting cross-legged remain extremely painful and impossible to maintain for long periods.

SHAKING

Violent shaking may be haphazard or, as in the case of Israel, systematic and planned. In such cases, bruising may be found on the chest or shoulders where the victim was seized but otherwise there are few outward signs. In the acute phase there is usually headache, disorientation and often a changed mental state. The most severe cases demonstrate all the features, potentially fatal, that have been well documented in shaken infant syndrome – cerebral oedema, subdural haematoma and retinal haemorrhage, the last being the major sign that makes possible a diagnosis before death. It has been named the shaken adult syndrome.[14]

BURNING

The application of heat is frequently employed by torturers. It produces immediate and long-term effects that are similar to those caused accidentally, but it is often possible to determine the deliberate nature of the injury if it is widely distributed in different parts of the body or if there are numerous similar lesions. For this reason it is important to take a detailed history in order to learn the nature of the agents used, the situation and posture of the subject and the duration of the application. Of course, if the victim was blindfolded or hooded during torture, he may not be able to describe the method of burning. In later cases, it is important to enquire as to the immediate effects and appearance of the wounds and how long they took to heal. If there was merely initial erythema or blistering and no infection supervened, it is likely that there will be no permanent scarring but if there was infection, sloughing and delay in healing for a month or more, recognisable scarring would be expected.

The pattern of scarring gives a clue to the method used. Flame burns caused by setting clothing alight leave different patterns from the application of blowlamps or other flames.

Caustic or acid burns may leave a trail indicating the victim's posture. Scarring tends to be more florid, perhaps with keloid formation than similarly-configured scars caused by scalding with boiling water.

Heated metal rods, branding irons or electrically heated devices such as smoothing irons or soldering irons often leave scars of distinctive shape and if they are multiple it makes accidental injury most unlikely.

Melted candle wax or plastic gives a characteristic pattern of scarring which indicates the flow of the hot liquid, and burning rubber tyres, etc. are placed round the neck in 'necklacing', leave burns over the whole upper body.

Cigarettes are particularly a common torture weapon. The scars they leave depend on the way the cigarettes were applied to the skin. If they were touched lightly or simply brushed against the skin they may leave no scar or something that is indistinguishable from a scar from acne, chicken pox or insect bite. On the other hand, if the cigarettes were deliberately stubbed out and held immobile on the skin, the scar is often characteristically circular about one centimetre in diameter, with a sharply demarcated pigmented periphery and a tissue paper centre, sometimes with an umbilicated appearance. The feature that makes it almost certain that the burns were deliberately inflicted is the presence of patterns on a part of the skin surface that the history indicates would be exposed. Thus, if the victim was strapped to a chair, there may be a line of scars on the knuckles, up the forearms or on the front of the thighs.

ASPHYXIATION

The commonest way of inducing asphyxia to near-death is *submarino* as it is nicknamed in Latin American countries. The head is immersed in water for minutes at a time to the point of drowning, then brought out and immersed again. In some countries the victim is suspended by the ankles and lowered repeatedly into a tank. A variant of *submarino* is for a plastic bag or similar impervious material filled with liquid to be tied over the head. In all these techniques the water is often contaminated with sewage or chemicals, adding to the immediate distress and increasing the likelihood of permanent ill-effects.

Dry submarino is practised with a plastic bag or similar impervious material placed over the head and tied tightly round the neck. Again, there is often contaminated material or an irritant such as chilli powder inside the bag. In Sri Lanka a small amount of petrol is often put in the bag[15] so that there is chemical poisoning as well as asphyxiation.

Chiffon is the name given to the method of asphyxiation used in Algeria.[16] Though details vary, it usually consists of the victim being held down on a bench and forced to take large amounts of water, often contaminated, into the mouth, most of which is swallowed while some is inevitably inhaled. A wedge may be put between the teeth or a rag may be stuffed into the mouth. This causes painful distension of the stomach as well as partial asphyxiation. After a great deal of liquid has been swallowed an officer may kick or punch the victim in the stomach, making him vomit.

The *immediate effects* of these techniques vary according to whether there has been any contamination. If so, there is likely to be severe upper respiratory and perhaps bronchopulmonary inflammation. Conjunctivitis or otitis media may follow, particularly after *submarino*. Irritants such as petrol or chilli may cause a dermatitis which is indistinguishable from acne. Any *long-term effects* of these techniques are not easy to assess but many victims attribute their asthma or bronchitis to have been asphyxiated many years previously. If there was no history of pre-existing disability, it may be reasonable to consider this as a possibility.

REFERENCES

1   Amnesty International. Take a Step to Stamp Out Torture. London: Amnesty International 2000
2   Medical Foundation for the Care of Victims of Torture. Guidelines for the Examination of Survivors of Torture, 2nd edn. Medical Foundation for the Care of Victims of Torture, 2000

3   Istanbul Protocol. See: Welsh J. The problem of torture, Chapter 1 in this book
4   Malik GH *et al.* Acute renal failure following physical torture. Nephron 1993; 63:434–437
5   Lok V *et al.* Bone scintigraphy as a clue to previous torture. Lancet 1991; 337:846–847
6   Mirzael S *et al.* Bone scintigraphy in screening of torture survivors. Lancet 1998; 352:949–951
7   Skylv G. Physical sequelae of torture. In: Basoglu M (ed.) Torture and its Consequences: Current Treatment Approaches. Cambridge: Cambridge University Press, 1992, pp 38–55
8   Rasmussen OV. Medical aspects of torture. Dan Med Bull 1990; 37(suppl 1):1–88
9   See: Lök V, Aytaclar S. Radiodiagnostic Approaches in the Documentation of Torture, Chapter 14 in this book
10 Savnik A, Amris K, Rogind H, *et al.* MRI of the plantar structures of the foot after falanga torture. Eur Radiol 2000; 10(10):1655–1659
11 Jempson M. Torture worldwide. In: Forrest D for Amnesty International (ed.) A Glimpse of Hell: Reports of Torture Worldwide. London: Cassell, 1996, pp 46–82
12 B'Tselem. Torture as a Routine: the Interrogation Methods of the GSS. Jerusalem: B'Tselem, 1998
13 Medical Foundation for the Care of Victims of Torture. Lives under Threat: a Study of Sikhs Coming to the UK from the Punjab, 2nd edn. Medical Foundation for the Care of Victims of Torture, 1999
14 Pounder D. Shaken adult syndrome. Am J Forensic Med Pathol 1997; 18:321–324
15 Medical Foundation for the Care of Victims of Torture. Caught in the Middle: A Study of Tamil Torture Survivors Coming to the UK from Sri Lanka. Medical Foundation for the Care of Victims of Torture, 2000, p 24
16 Peel M. Failure to protect: survivors of torture from Algeria. Medical Foundation for the Care of Victims of Torture, London, 1999. Available on: http://www. torturecare.org.uk/pubbrf6.htm

11

THE SEXUAL ABUSE
OF FEMALES

Gill Hinshelwood

INTRODUCTION

In 1999, 33% of asylum seekers coming to the UK were women. The majority were single men; some were accompanied by wife and children. Once these men had begun to feel a little safer, their thoughts were on the relatives (wives, partners, children, parents and siblings) and friends they had left behind. What did they expect would happen to them? It has taken time for host countries to recognise that women, either accompanied by their male kin, or unaccompanied, also have experiences to recount of persecution and torture. They are mostly reluctant to speak at length, or at all, of their experiences. At immigration, solicitors, or even in the doctor's surgery they may have been interviewed in the presence of male members of their family, or ignored. Alone, they find the presence of a male immigration officer or interpreter inhibiting, and even if the interpreter is female, if she is of the same nationality as the asylum seeker she may well be mistrusted to keep confidence. Only in a minority of cases do the women claim to be politically active, or are able to describe just why they fear it would be dangerous to return. It is often many months or years before some women will reveal that they have been singled out and sexually abused, most commonly because the police or army are seeking their husband, father, or son.

It has been found in Chile,[1] and by health care volunteers for Amnesty International that taking a detailed testimony from torture survivors can be a highly therapeutic process. The second important discovery was that torture survivors seem to be particularly unable to access the health and social service benefits to which they are entitled in their host country.[2] It is important to keep these two findings in mind when women are referred for medical reports to document their torture. First and foremost the consultation should be a meaningful experience for the patient, a therapeutic opportunity.

HISTORY TAKING

The request for a medical report usually comes from a lawyer representing an immigration application or a criminal investigation, or from a Human Rights organisation, for example Amnesty International. Sometimes the lawyer has taken a full history of general persecution, events leading up to the arrest, detention and torture, and history of escape and flight. Experience of abuse and torture may take up only a paragraph of the whole statement. It is the doctor's responsibility to concentrate on the physical and psychological violence to which the woman was subjected. Most doctors like to set this in context for themselves, and build up a picture of their patient's life. Some doctors proceed chronologically from the time of the first physical or verbal assault, others prefer to start with the present. The woman should be asked to bring any medication she is currently taking, and the name and address of her doctor and any specialist she is or has been attending. It is important that doctor and interpreter are both women. The purpose of the interview needs to be explained, and the doctor must be satisfied that the woman really understands why she is being interviewed and examined. It is helpful if the doctor indicates the extent of the correspondence she has had with the referrer relating to the woman. This usually includes a letter, and in asylum cases, the woman's political asylum questionnaire, and a statement that she has made some time in the past. A medical report may be requested days or weeks after the torture, or up to 10 or more years after the event.

Starting at the present gives a frightened or troubled woman a sense that someone is interested in her and helps to create a situation of trust. It also gives an idea of the woman's preoccupations about her health and to what factors she may attribute her symptoms and problems.

Sometimes starting with the present leads straight to the past. Mrs Rosa A's main complaint was pain around both shoulders. When she was asked more about this, how long it had been present, what she thought was the cause of it, she described clearly how her arms were wrenched behind her and she was pushed and pulled by a number of soldiers all fighting for their turn to rape her. On other occasions the present problems, such as housing and poverty, dominate. Ms Marcia B's main concern was the mental state of her son, a toddler of two years, who cried a great deal and in general did not seem to thrive. Exploration of this led to a discussion of her ambivalence towards this child. It took a while before she was able to say that he had been the result of a rape. When taking a history of the events leading up to the assault, observe where the woman wants to start. Sometimes she gives a wealth of generalisations, about ideology, persecution, what happened to other people. Is this because she is delaying the dreadful moments, when she has to put the unspeakable into words, or, are there no particulars? Is it because this is what most questioners have wanted to know? It may be helpful to wonder about this with her. It is important to stress that details of her own experience are required, show interest in what happened to her, and emphasise that the task is to build up a picture of the physical and mental experiences to which she was subjected.

The history of the assault, or assaults should be explored in detail. Women often say 'then I fainted' after being knocked to the floor, or having their clothes dragged from them. The doctor needs to be encouragingly persistent at this point. How much violence? How many men? How was she held down? Ms Carla C was a student leader of a campaign for women's rights in a repressive regime. Intimidation and harassment gradually increased in intensity, over months, and she and her group became more determined and united in their efforts. But she was very unprepared for the first night in custody after being arrested from a demonstration. She was held in a small cell, alone. She had been questioned for what seemed like hours, deprived of food and water, and slapped about the face, kicked and verbally threatened and abused. In the night about five policemen dragged her into another, larger room, tore off her clothes and raped her one by one. They were drinking alcohol and smoking. She became hysterical and started screaming and shouting, and one of them pushed a dirty rag into her mouth. They tried to force her to drink alcohol, and when she refused they tried to force oral sex on her. They scratched the inside of her thighs forcing her legs apart, and touched their lighted cigarettes on her arms and legs. They sucked and bit her breasts. They left her exhausted, collapsed on the floor, and messy with semen and blood drying on her. During the assault a bottle had broken, and as Ms C took in what had happened to her she felt so vile and shamed she cut her wrist with a shard of glass. She was discovered and taken to be stitched up (without an anaesthetic), and warned not to tell anyone what had happened to her.

EXAMINATION

Privacy must be ensured. It is always helpful to have the interpreter present, but both patient and interpreter prefer to be screened off. This may well be the examination the woman has wanted for a long time, but been unable to request. Note posture, and comfort sitting in the chair. Throughout the interview note respiration, the presence or absence of shallow breathing, overbreathing, sweating, and tremor. Ask her to extend her hands to check for tremor, and ask the handedness. Take her blood pressure and pulse. Then it is appropriate to suggest to the woman that examination begins at the top of her head, working downwards. Ask about blows to the head and face, whether wounds bled, if there was bruising, how long did it last. Inquire about hearing, or discharge from the ears, and examine them if necessary. Move down the body slowly, looking at neck movements and shoulder movements. Frequently women complain of pain in this region, as in our above example. Examine both arms, taking note of vaccination marks, and more recent lesions, such as caused by cooking accidents. Some women will volunteer that they are more forgetful these days, and burn themselves on the stove. Look for signs of self-harm around the wrists. Note all lesions and how the woman says she has come by them. It is kind to suggest that one part of the body be covered when the examination is over, before moving on to the next area. Examine the breasts. Some women volunteer that they were mauled around, hit or bitten. Bites frequently become infected, so a lesion is likely to be present, but most scratches and bruises will have healed. However, it is important to ask what was present immediately after the attack, and what the woman did about it.

Many women give a history of being beaten across the back, or hit in the abdomen. Examine for lash marks, and marks from other forms of beating, for example, with the butt of a gun. Note the care of the skin, is it dry, are there many old healed infected spots? Can these be attributed to infestations in prison, or past acne scars? Palpate the abdomen, looking for tenderness, or tensing of muscles. Note any operation scars and stretch marks.

It is a good idea to encourage the woman to take off her lower garments and lie on the couch at this point. Here, in a good light, the legs can be examined for lesions, and for musculoskeletal disorders.[3] Many women report being kicked, and a severe kick from a soldier's boot on the shin can leave a circular depressed scar. Kicking and beating on the legs can give rise to irregular patches of pigmented and depigmented areas, especially over the bone. Running through forest to escape also may give rise to lesions on the lower legs, especially the fronts. Sexual violence may give rise to lesions on the inner thighs, where women have had their legs forced apart. These may be scratches, cigarette burns, knife wounds.[4]

The vaginal examination is then conducted, taking note of the labia, the presence or absence of vaginismus, the presence or absence of a hymen, the possibility of previous pregnancies, discharge, tenderness. Note if the woman has been subjected to female genital mutilation. Examine the anus if the woman has indicated that anal sex was performed. In this area of the body, which has previously been penetrated without consent, it is important to describe exactly what you intend to do, and what is found. Explain carefully that this examination is not a test for sexually transmitted diseases, and that tests for these can be discussed when the examination is over. The vaginal examination has been described by doctors who have trained with the Institute of Psychosexual Medicine as 'the moment of truth'. This is not to be used in the medicolegal sense of the phrase. At her most vulnerable, a woman's emotions are more easily accessible and the sensitive doctor can respond in a therapeutic way. Ms Soraya D became increasingly anxious as the examination proceeded. Already she had said that her periods were normal and that STD clinic had found no sign of infection. Her distress was remarked on. 'Will I be able to have children?' she sobbed. The soldiers who raped her said they had damaged her so that would be one less Tutsi brat in the world. On the other hand, the 'moment of truth' sometimes is of medicolegal importance. Ms Esther E had made a statement that she had no children. She was very afraid of being examined. I saw why. She had extensive abdominal striae. When confronted with this her fear gave way to grief. She had fled leaving three children with her mother. She had no news. She dreamed about them all night. This woman became 'real' for the first time in the consultation. Of course it meant starting all over again with the history.

PSYCHOLOGICAL ISSUES

During the history taking something of the woman's past and present mental state will be revealed. How she lives, the visits to her GP and the medication she has been prescribed are important indicators. Her sociability and level of English after a certain time in the UK (if it is a second language) suggest her ability to function in the present, and this can be compared with a history of her past attainments. Mrs Aleyna F aged 23 years had a carrier bag full of bottles of pills, creams and hospital appointment cards. She had been given ever stronger inhalers and antibiotics for nocturnal breathlessness and sweating, painkillers, and antacids. She described insomnia 'but really I'm afraid to go to sleep. I see the men over and over again, and I'm unable to escape'. She also described daytime flashbacks of events that had happened to her, panics in a crowd, mood swings and forgetfulness about day to day activities. She was suffering from many of the symptoms of post-traumatic stress disorder.[5] A Rape Trauma Syndrome has also been described.[6]

One particularly valuable approach is to consider the crisis emotions and how they present in patients. The crisis emotions are fear, anger, grief and shame. Even though many of the patients that are referred for medical reports have been in the UK for a few years, it is unlikely that these emotions have resolved completely. Their presence is a huge barrier to the recovery of stable mental functioning. They are also indicators of the nature of the assault.

Fear is what drives the woman to flee. Many women describe months or years of harassment before leaving their country. Ms C cited above, put up with taunts, being given poor marks in class, and being singled out and threatened by her tutors. But her rapes in prison, and the threats of worse violence drove her to leave. It was fear which made it impossible for her to sleep at night. With the light and her radio full on she whiled away the nights, terrified that the police would track her down and kill her.

It may take time before the extent of anger that a survivor carries is apparent. To express it may only be possible once safety is assured. Mrs Farah F wanted revenge. Every muscle of her body ached and she swallowed many painkillers each day, and had endless medical consultations and opinions. It seemed as if all her anger was stored up in her taut and fatigued body. She plotted every night, unrealistically, to return one day to her country and single-handedly kill her torturer.

Grief may be a much more visible emotion, some women displaying it abundantly, while others endeavour to keep it in check, often to the point of presenting in a cool and rather detached manner. The doctor was alerted to the grief of a very emotionless woman when she herself was feeling quite distressed, then turned to her interpreter to find tears streaming down her face. When this was talked through with the patient, she revealed how she felt that if she once allowed herself to cry or even feel the sadness, she would drown in tears for there was nothing else in her.

Shame has been called 'the Cinderella of emotions'.[7] When a woman is raped or otherwise sexually abused, the perpetrator knows that he has inflicted very severe harm to her. The shame may lead some women to kill themselves, or attempt to. The medicolegal examination is an opportunity to observe, and to discuss therapeutically, the pernicious damaging effects of shame. Miss Theresa G missed two appointments and arrived late for the third. She sat making very little eye contact. Her statement had been bland in the extreme. In it she had stated that she had been arrested from the market square where she had been demonstrating. She had been beaten up, locked up, and then four men had attempted to rape her, but she had screamed and they backed off. This had not been the doctor's prior experience of reports from this woman's country. The doctor put it to Miss G that she was not behaving like a woman who could fight off assailants. Then the real violence of the rape she had been subjected to emerged, and Miss G was able to show the scars on the inside of her legs, and talk about her abdominal pain for the first time. Miss G had been living in isolation in a small room, afraid of meeting anyone lest they could tell, just by looking at her, that she was a 'soiled' woman. She never looked in a mirror, for fear of what she might see.

Women, of course, do present with other emotions. They feel guilty for leaving children behind, worry about elderly parents, and bitterness about their change in circumstances. However, in the presence of any one or more of the crisis emotions the responsibility of the doctor is to explore and document the crises to which they relate.

Women refugees are the most vulnerable population group in whatever country they seek refuge. Nevertheless, with a little help they can also prove to be highly resourceful and resilient. Medically examining them and documenting their torture is an important part of the help they need and can use.

REFERENCES

1   Cienfugos AJ, Monelli C. The testimony of political repression as a therapeutic instrument. Am J Orthopsych 1983; 53(1): 43–51
2   Jones D, Gill PS. Refugees and primary care: tackling the inequalities. BMJ 1998; 317:1444–1446
3   See: Kirschner R, Peel M. Physical examination for late signs of torture, Chapter 9 in this book
4   Howitt J, Rogers D. Adult sexual offences and related matters. In: McLay WDS (ed.), Clinical Forensic Medicine. London: Greenwich Medical Media, 1996, pp 193–218
5   See: Allden K. The psychological consequences of torture, Chapter 7 in this book
6   Burgess AW, Holdstrom LL. Rape trauma syndrome. Am J Psychiatry 1974; 131:981–986
7   Rycroft C. Psychoanalysis Observed. London: Penguin, 1968

12

MALE SEXUAL ABUSE
IN DETENTION

Michael Peel

INTRODUCTION

It is widely accepted that women in detention are regularly sexually assaulted and raped as a form of torture, and that in some countries the rape of women in detention by their guards is routine.[1] There is also literature about the rape of men in prisons by other prisoners as part of the power hierarchy,[2] although the frequency of this is unclear.[3] However, what has rarely been studied is the sexual assault and rape of male detainees by their guards or interrogators.[4,5] This chapter describes a study of medical reports that were written by doctors at the Medical Foundation for the Care of Victims of Torture in London about male patients referred in the period 1 January 1997 to 30 June 1998. These reports were written in support of asylum claims on patients referred to the Medical Foundation by their solicitor when, in the expert opinion of the doctor, the patient had been tortured as he described. Some patients are seen a few months after their torture, but most come several years later. Those whose alleged torture prior to 1992 were excluded from the study. Thus the data reflect torture practices around the world over the last decade. However, patients come to the UK and the Medical Foundation for specific reasons, and the relative numbers do not reflect the prevalence of torture in the various countries.

RESULTS

Medical reports were written on a total of 607 men from 45 countries, of whom 153 (25.2%) had been sexually assaulted in detention by their guards or interrogators, including 33 (5.4%) who had been raped. Sexual assaults were categorised as

- assaults to the genitals;
- electric shocks to the genitals and anus;
- object inserted in the urethral meatus;
- object inserted through the anus;
- rape;
- forced sexual acts.

Thirty-two men had been tortured in two or more of these ways.

On examination, only 34 of the 153 men who had been sexually assaulted had any physical signs relating to the sexual part of the torture (22.2%). Thus in 119 men who had been sexually assaulted (77.8%) there were no relevant physical signs.

About half of the men in the sample were assaulted directly on the genitals, although this included a wide variety of forms of torture. Sixteen were kicked in the genitals, and 11 were hit with batons and sticks. Other forms of torture included the penis being pulled, sometimes with some string or wire tied around it first (seven men), weights being hung on the scrotum (two men), the genitals being put in a heavy desk drawer which was slammed shut (two men), pins or needles being pushed into the penis (two men); one man had chillies rubbed into his genitals, and one had his penis squeezed until it burst. Four men had their penis or scrotum cut, and six men were burnt on the genitals, two with cigarettes, one with a match, one with a burning stick, one with hot metal, and one with boiling water. Many of the men did not know exactly what had happened to them, as they had been blindfolded during the torture.

Forty-one men were subjected to electric shocks to the genitals and/or the anus, only two of whom had any physical signs. One was a man from North Cyprus who had four small scars on the glans of his penis from the clips through which the electric shocks had been administered. The other was an Indian man who had narrowing of his urethral meatus following electric shocks to the tip of his penis. It is significant to note that electric shocks were used as the principal means of sexual torture in India and Turkey, where there is a degree of judicial independence and the police are perhaps more careful than in some other countries not to leave scars.

Of the 73 men who were assaulted on the genitals, 20 (27.4%) had some physical signs. Not surprisingly, all the four men who were cut and four of the six men who were burnt had recognisable scarring, as did the man whose penis burst when it was squeezed. Both the men whose penis was trapped in a drawer had scarring related to the incident. Three of the men who were pulled by the penis had physical signs. One had a circular scar around the penis where the wire had cut in, one had an irregular piece of foreskin missing where the string had pulled it away, and the other had been circumcised subsequent to the event, but no contemporaneous medical records were available to support the history. Of the ones who had been hit with sticks, two had non-specific scars. These findings by themselves would not be considered evidence of torture, but following the overall examination of the patient, they were thought to be significant (Table 12.1).

Most of the men tortured by objects being introduced into the urethra were from Nigeria, where the twig of the broom plant was often used. Three of the eight men who had been tortured by objects inside the penis had relevant physical findings. Two had palpable thickening of the urethra. The third was being held in a British Immigration Detention Centre where he was complaining of difficulty on passing urine. He had some tenderness of the urethra, but no discharge. The doctor employed by the Detention Centre kept treating him for a sexually transmitted disease, apparently because he was Nigerian, even though the history of sexual abuse was well documented and there was no suggestion that the patient had ever put himself at risk of contracting a sexually transmitted disease. Only when the patient was referred to the local hospital was his history taken seriously and he was found to have urethral damage on cystoscopy. The operation had to be performed under general anaesthetic because it was far too distressing for the patient to be aware of the cystoscope being

Table 12.1

Country	No. of patients	No. of sexually abused	% of sexually abused	Assault to genitals	Electric shocks	Object in meatus	Object in anus	Rape	Forced sexual activity
Algeria	11	5	45.5	3	1	0	3	1	0
Angola	27	7	25.9	2	0	0	1	4	1
Cameroon	17	2	11.8	2	0	0	0	0	1
India	56	12	21.4	3	9	0	1	0	0
Iran	37	6	16.2	4	0	1	1	0	0
Iraq	21	9	42.9	1	6	0	1	0	0
Kenya	20	10	50.0	7	1	0	3	2	0
Nigeria	51	14	27.5	7	0	5	2	3	0
Pakistan	14	4	28.6	3	0	0	2	0	0
Sri Lanka	137	26	19.0	14	3	1	3	9	5
Sudan	19	9	47.4	4	2	0	2	3	0
Turkey	65	17	26.2	7	12	1	2	0	0
Zaire/DRC	37	10	27.0	3	2	0	3	5	1
Europe	13	3	23.1	1	1	0	0	1	0
North Africa	18	5	27.8	4	1	0	0	0	0
Other Africa	45	8	17.8	5	0	0	0	3	0
Other Asia	7	1	14.3	1	0	0	0	0	0
Other Middle East	12	5	41.7	2	2	0	1	1	0
Total	607	153	25.2	73	41	8	25	32	8
% abused				47.7	26.8	5.2	16.3	20.9	5.2
Physical findings				20	2	3	5	4	0
% with physical findings				27.4	4.9	37.5	20.0	12.5	0.0

Europe: Bulgaria, North Cyprus, Romania, Russia, Ukraine, former Yugoslavia.
North Africa: Eritrea, Ethiopia, Libya, Morocco, Somalia, Tunisia.
Other Africa: Congo (Brazzaville), Gambia, Ghana, Ivory Coast, Rwanda, Sierra Leone, South Africa, Tanzania, Togo, Uganda, Zimbabwe.
Other Asia: Afghanistan, China, Myanmar (Burma), Nepal.
Other Middle East: Bahrain, Egypt, Lebanon, Syria, Yemen.

inserted in his penis. Perhaps other patients might have physical findings on cystoscopy, but it would be unethical to examine them in this way without any clinical indication.

Five of the 25 men who had objects inserted in the anus (20.0%) and four of the 32 men who had been raped (12.5%) were noted to have physical signs. These include one man who had non-specific scarring around the anus following a truncheon being inserted, then being raped. Eight of the men had bottles pushed through their anus, one of whom was left with significant scarring around the anus. In North Africa, this takes the form of making a man squat naked with the top of a bottle pushed into his anus, then pushing him and kicking him so that he loses balance and the wider part of the bottle enters and stretches his anus. Seven men had truncheons and batons pushed through their anus, two of whom being left with perianal scarring including the man noted above. A Nigerian man had an umbrella pushed through his anus and opened up. The pain made him lose consciousness, and he was left with substantial scarring. Two Sri Lankan men had sticks covered with chilli paste pushed through their anus. Three men had hoses pushed through, two of whom had water poured into the rectum, the third had diesel inserted and he was left with a perianal irritation around the anus several years later which he attributed to the incident. One man who had been raped on a large number of occasions was noted by the examining doctor to have a lax anal sphincter. Another man who had been raped was noted to have a small anal skin tag. An African man was HIV positive, which he attributed to being raped in detention. Thus most of the anal signs were thought to be significant by the examining doctors.

Of the eight men who were forced to perform sexual acts, five were raped orally and one was made to masturbate a soldier manually, five of these six were Sri Lankan. One African was made to have intercourse with a female dog. The other African gave a story of a woman having been put in the cell with him and having sex with him. He subsequently found out that he had contracted a sexually transmitted disease, and he believes that the authorities put her into the cell with him in order to infect him. None of these eight men had any relevant physical findings.

Patterns of abuse

Male sexual abuse must be seen in the context of detention and torture. It takes very many forms, some of which are widespread. At least three patterns can be identified. In the first, which could be considered the Nigerian pattern, the sexual abuse seems to have been part of the overall pattern of brutality. The taboos that appear to exist in most parts of the world about the penis are not present. Inserting the twig of a broom plant into the penis is just another way of causing agony as part of what the torturer calls an interrogation.[6]

In the second, which could be considered the Algerian pattern, male sexual abuse was part of the process of intimidation of the community by the security services. The release of semi-conscious and severely beaten individuals was intended to discourage any form of protest.[7] Anal abuse and rape of men was intended to add to this by maximising the humiliation as well as the pain of the torture. It was made known to the community that men who had been detained in police stations would have been sexually assaulted, and should no longer have the status of males in the community.[8]

In the third, which could be considered the Sri Lankan pattern, the majority of the sexual abuse in detention is, as everywhere else, a part of the torture. However, the rape is not. The men generally describe a drunken soldier coming into their cell in the evening, either alone or with one or two colleagues. The man is then taken to the soldier's quarters where he is raped,[5] and sometimes he is also made to perform other sexual acts. The detainee is therefore treated as a prize. One victim, who had been detained for a number of years, said that he was given for sexual purposes to visitors to the military camp. Another said that the rapes generally did not happen when senior officers were around; the junior officers raped any female detainees, leaving the other ranks their choice of the male detainees.

Psychological impact

As part of the study, an analysis was made of the psychological symptoms described by the men. In total, 224 of the 607 men (37%) described a pattern of symptoms consistent with post-traumatic stress disorder,[9] including difficulty getting to sleep, nightmares, flashbacks, jumpiness and irritability, behaviour to avoid being reminded of the abuse, and depression. Some 121 men described most but not all of these symptoms, and 138 described sleep disorders but not the other symptoms. The other 124 men said that they had no psychological symptoms, although some of these might have chosen not to talk about these symptoms, and others might not have fully understood the concept of psychological symptoms. However, the percentage is similar to the first main study of female rape, in which 14% of the women did not complain of symptoms[10] (Table 12.2).

What is remarkable is that 36.9% of all the men who had been tortured were suffering from the symptoms of post-traumatic stress disorder. This proportion increases to 55.8% of the men who had been sexually assaulted in detention, and 71.9% of the

Table 12.2

Psychological symptoms	None	Sleep	Many	PTSD
Raped	4 (12.5%)	4 (12.5%)	1 (3.1%)	23 (71.9%)
All sexually abused	19 (12.3%)	26 (16.9%)	23 (14.9%)	86 (55.8%)
Not abused	105 (23.2%)	112 (24.7%)	98 (21.6%)	138 (30.5%)
Total	124 (20.4%)	138 (22.7%)	121 (19.9%)	224 (36.9%)

Table 12.3

Country	Prevalence of PTSD symptoms	
	Raped (%)	Not raped (%)
All	71.9	35.0
Angola	75.0	30.4
Sri Lanka	66.7	22.7
Zaire/DRC	60.0	31.3

men who had been raped. This emphasises the particular psychological trauma of sexual assault and rape in detention. In case these results are caused by the nationality of the victims of rape, the analysis was repeated for the three countries from which the largest numbers of rape victims came. The results are given in Table 12.3.

DISCUSSION

In this study of victims of torture, more than a quarter of men detained by the security services were sexually assaulted, varying from just over 11% in Cameroon to 50% in Kenya. Lunde and Ortmann[4] found that 56% of the men in their sample had been sexually abused, although their sample was dominated by men from Latin America and the Middle East, whereas the current study has no men from Latin America. For many countries, the numbers were too small to analyse individually. However, it is clear that where torture of men exists, a significant proportion of them will have a sexual component to that torture. Torture is one of the greatest taboos in societies, as is sexual assault, so it is not surprising that those who break one may have no scruples in breaking the other. All clinicians dealing with male victims of torture must be aware that there could have been a sexual component.

More than 5% of the men were raped by their guards, being about 20% of all the men who were sexually tortured. In some countries, such as Angola and Zaire/DRC, rape was reported relatively frequently. In others, such as Iran and Iraq, it was not reported at all, although it is not clear whether this is lack of reporting for cultural reasons, or because male detainees were not raped. However, in most countries the number of victims of torture seen was too small to establish whether male rape was or was not a significant issue, but there is no evidence to suggest that the incidence of rape is different to that of sexual torture generally.

Of the men who were sexually assaulted, 22% had physical signs of the assault. However, only 4.9% of the men who had been given electric shocks to the genitals had any physical signs. In this particular population this finding was not so important, as most of the men had physical signs from their non-sexual torture. However, this finding reinforces the fact that the absence of physical signs does not imply that torture has not occurred.

Some 27.4% of those who were beaten on the genitals has physical signs. However, it is important to recognise that the skin of the penis and scrotum is difficult to damage and generally heals without scarring, so any scars present must be the result of severe injury.[11] Of the men who were kicked, one had an atrophied testis. A large study of victims of torture included six men with testicular atrophy that had not been apparent before torture, out of 41 who had been beaten severely in the genitals (14.6%).[12]

In 12.9% of the men who were raped, and in 16.3% of the men who had objects inserted in the anus there were physical signs. Mostly these were perianal scars. Scarring from anal fissures is seen in a proportion of the general population, but an experienced examining doctor can give an opinion that the scarring seen is either in an unusual location or larger than that normally seen following anal fissures.[13] Where an object has been inserted through the anus which causes significant bleeding for several days, there might be internal damage, but not otherwise. A lax anal sphincter can be found after repeated anal intercourse,[14] and this was found in one case of a man who had been raped repeatedly over a prolonged period.

History and examination

Following a more general history, questions should be asked about urinary function after the episode(s). In one study, 16% of male victims of torture described haematuria for a median of two days, mostly after beating or electric shocks to the genitals, although a few could have had haemaglobinuria from beatings elsewhere in the body.[12] Where an object has been inserted into the anus, including anal rape, there is normally bleeding and pain for a few days afterwards, but these symptoms do not last for more than about two weeks.[12] Following rape the other issue is sexually transmitted diseases, for example a history of rectal discharge is obviously significant.

An opportunity should be given to the patient to describe sexual problems, especially if he has a wife or other regular sexual partner. However, if a man has had some unsuccessful attempts at sexual activity, he may not want to disclose this, even to a doctor. If he has left a wife and family behind, and comes from a society which takes a punitive attitude to extramarital sexual activity, he will be particularly unwilling to disclose it. Some men will have had difficulties masturbating and will be concerned about this, both for itself and for the possibility of a normal marital relationship in due course. Again they need to be given reassurance, whether they disclose their problem or not.

Victims of sexual assault in detention are rarely released from detention when acute lesions are present. Where they are, the lesions should be documented in detail and, where possible, photographed.[15] Following rape, samples should be taken from the rectum for gonorrhoea and chlamydia, and also air dried internal and external anal swabs for DNA testing up to five days after the rape if there is any possibility of the perpetrator being prosecuted, even if the victim has defecated since the rape.

The examination of the patient alleging a sexual part to his torture is not technically different from a general anogenital examination of a male. The essential aspect, even more than for other medical purposes, is to gain the confidence of the individual. By this stage the doctor will have already completed an interview and general physical examination. Sometimes it is better to leave the history of sexual abuse and the anogenital examination to a subsequent interview, if this is possible. However, other patients prefer to complete the examination in a single session, not wanting to wait knowing they will have an intimate examination.

For the majority of patients, simple visual examination of the anogenital region is sufficient. The doctor should look for scarring and other lesions of the skin, the focus of the inspection being guided by the history. Scars on the penis are often quite small, so it is necessary to inspect it in detail where there is a history of electric shocks, burns or cuts, particularly under the prepuce if the patient is uncircumcised. Small scars, for example from electrode clips, may be seen in the folds of the scrotum. The insides of the thighs may also be the site of scarring. The anus is best examined in the left lateral position,[14] the buttocks being pulled apart gently to look for perianal scarring. Digital examination of the anal sphincter may be appropriate in a man who has been raped repeatedly over a prolonged period. Only if there is a history of substantial bleeding following an object being inserted through the anus, and the patient is willing, proctoscopy can be performed.

Psychological aspects

Many men do not easily disclose the fact that there had been a sexual component to their torture. In most of the cases in the study this is not essential to their asylum claim, because they had sufficient evidence of non-sexual torture for a medicolegal report to be written supporting their assertion of torture. Therapeutically, the situation is very different. Many men were making little progress until the clinician raised the possibility of sexual abuse. Once the matter had been discussed, they then started making significant progress. The major reason why the men did not disclose it was shame.

Several victims of rape described guilt at not fighting off their assailants, as is also described by female rape victims.[16] When it was pointed out to them that resistance would have been impossible in the situation, the patients readily agreed, but on subsequent discussion the brooding about acquiescence had continued.

Some men are accused by the British immigration authorities of having fabricated a history of rape because they did not express emotion when describing abuse. However, all studies of rape victims, male and female, show a significant percentage of victims having a calm, composed or subdued affect when interviewed about the rape.[10,17]

Men who have been tortured sexually are often told as part of the torture that they will never be able to function sexually again. This can become a self-fulfilling prophecy.

Additionally, when a man embarks on voluntary sexual activity, he may well get flash-backs of his sexual torture or feelings of guilt and shame, and these will impede his sexual function, for example causing impotence or premature ejaculation.[18]

Men who have been anally abused in detention, and particularly those who have been raped, are frequently concerned about their sexuality.[18] It is a physiological reaction for a man to have an erection, and sometimes ejaculate, both because of the emotional arousal from anger, fear and pain.[19] They, too, need to be reassured that such a response will happen in a man who is heterosexual, and need not interfere with their preferred sexual activity. This stress is exacerbated when the man is not believed because of these false notions. This is particularly true when detainees have been forced to rape each other, because many people believe erroneously that a man cannot become sufficiently aroused to have intercourse against his will.

In order to be able to reassure men that such responses are normal, the clinician must be aware that sexual abuse and rape in detention are not uncommon in many countries from which refugees come, but that the patient is often unwilling to discuss the episode or his fears. In time, and with help, it is possible for men who have been sexually assaulted or raped in detention to regain normal sexual function,[18] and the process starts by being able to acknowledge the experience.

Legal aspects

It does not need to be stressed that rape in detention is torture in that it is the deliberate infliction of severe physical or psychological pain, aggravated by the guard having complete control over the victim.

It is sometimes said that rape in detention is not torture because the guard is doing it for his own pleasure, and not to punish, intimidate or coerce.[20] However, it is widely recognised that rape is an attack dominated by feelings of power and anger, rather than being an expression of sexual desire.[21] Perpetrators of male rape generally do not perceive themselves by their actions to be homosexual.[2]

It is also sometimes said that rape in detention is not torture because it is not official policy, although no government now admits to torture being official policy. The fact that it is widespread in many countries, as shown by this paper, means that individual officials should be aware that it is happening, and if they are not aware, they are negligent.[22] Even when senior officers are not present, for example as described by a survivor from Sri Lanka, but are considered to be aware that the abuse is happening,[5] they must do everything in their power to stop it.

Although it was not analysed in detail in the study, there were cases of victims being raped by other prisoners with guards aware of and condoning the rapes. Generally this was in the context of the victim being a member of an ethnic minority and the other prisoners and the guards being from the majority, for example in Sri Lanka. However, this was not always the case. In Nigeria, for example, the rape was just part of the endemic violence by which the more brutal prisoners, generally with criminal convictions, establish their supremacy in the inmate hierarchy. The guards are either also intimidated by the violent prisoners, or are content to permit the hierarchy to persist because it makes their work easier. Clearly this fits into the UN Convention against Torture definition of torture in that it is inflicted with the acquiescence of a public official. It certainly cannot be argued that the suffering arises incidental to lawful sanctions.[20]

CONCLUSION

Sexual abuse in detention is torture. Sexual abuse of males is happening too commonly in many countries of the world. Men who have been sexually tortured, and particularly those who have been raped, find it difficult to disclose, principally because of shame. Relevant physical signs were seen in only 20% of all men who had been sexually tortured, and in only 12% of those who had been raped. Some 56% of those who had been sexually tortured and 72% of those who had been raped described all the symptoms of post-traumatic stress disorder, compared to 23% of those whose torture had not been sexual. This sexual torture causes much hidden distress, and the first stage of treating it is an awareness that any man who has been detained in a country where torture occurs could have suffered a sexual aspect to that torture.

Rape is not an act of personal sexual gratification but of power, and those who abuse positions in the prison service, security agencies, police and army must be punished. Men are often raped in detention to punish, to coerce confessions and to intimidate communities. Those in positions of authority in these countries must recognise that they have a role in preventing these widespread abuses. If they cannot demonstrate that they have done everything in their power to prevent sexual torture and rape in the prisons, police stations and army barracks under their control, they are guilty of a crime against humanity.[22]

REFERENCES

1 Man N. Children, Torture and Power. London: Save the Children Fund, 2000
2 Sagarin E. Prison homosexuality and its effect on post-prison sexual behaviour. Psychiatry 1976; 39:245–257
3 King MB. Male rape in institutional settings. In: Mezey G, King MB (eds), Male Victims of Sexual Assault. Oxford: Oxford University Press, 1992, pp 67–74
4 Lunde I, Ortmann J. Prevalence and sequelae of sexual torture. Lancet 1990 (4 August); 336:289–291
5 Peel M, Mahtani A, Hinshelwood G, Forrest D. The sexual abuse of men in detention in Sri Lanka. Lancet 2000; 355:2069–2070
6 Soyinka W. Ten years after. In: Soyinka W (ed.), The Man Died: Prison Notes. Ibadan: Spectrum Books, 1972; pp vii–xxiii

7   Algeria: fear and silence: a hidden human rights crisis. November 1996 AI Index: MDE 28/11/96

8   Peel M. Failure to protect: survivors of torture from Algeria. Medical Foundation for the Care of Victims of Torture. London, 1999. Available at: http://www.torturecare.org.uk/pubbrf6.htm

9   See: Allden K. The psychological consequences of torture, Chapter 7 in this book

10 Burgess AW, Holdstrom LL. Rape trauma syndrome. Am J Psychiatry 1974; 131:981–986

11 Peel M, Hinshelwood G, Forrest D. The physical and psychological findings following the late examination of victims of torture. Torture 2000; 10(1):12–15

12 Rasmussen OV. Medical aspects of torture. Dan Med Bull 1990; 37(suppl 1):1–88

13 Howitt J, Rogers D. Adult sexual offences and related matters. In: McLay WDS (ed.), Clinical Forensic Medicine. London: Greenwich Medical Media, 1996, pp 193–218

14 Goh B. The genitalia and sexually transmitted diseases. In: Swash M (ed.), Hutchinson's Clinical Methods. London: W.B. Saunders Company Ltd., 1995, pp 399–410

15 See: Ozkalipci O. Physical examination following allegations of recent torture, Chapter 8 in this book

16 Mezey GC, Taylor PJ. Psychological reactions of women who have been raped: a descriptive and comparative study. Br J Psychiatry 1988; 152:330–339

17 Kaufman A, Divasto P *et al.* Male rape victims: noninstitutionalised assault. Am J Psychiatry 1980; 137:221–223

18 van der Veer G. Counselling and Therapy with Refugees and Victims of Trauma. West Sussex: Wiley 1999, pp 141–150

19 Groth AN, Burgess AW. Male rape: offenders and victims. Am J Psychiatry 1980; 137:806–810

20 See: Welsh J. The problem of torture, Chapter 1 in this book

21 Groth AN, Burgess AW, Holdstrom LL. Rape: power, anger and sexuality. Am J Psychiatry 1977; 134:1239–1243

22 Rome Statute of International Criminal Court, Article 28

13

THE EXAMINATION AND INVESTIGATION OF ELECTRIC SHOCK INJURIES

Lis Danielsen

DEVICES

Use of electric torture has been frequently reported in the past decades.[1-11] Three sorts of devices are used in most or all cases, such as hand-cranked generators, mains current, and battery powered devices.

Hand-cranked magnetos were developed for use in field telephones in military operations, and were probably first used for torture in the Second World War.[12] They were used by the French in Algeria in the late 1950s,[1,13] and they have been used in many parts of the world since. They produce a relatively low DC current that increases in intensity when the handle is turned more quickly.

'In the hands of my torturers I saw a different machine, larger than the first, and in my very agony I felt the difference in quality. Instead of the sharp and rapid spasms that seemed to tear my body in two, it was now a greater pain that took possession of all my muscles and tightened them in longer spasms.'

Turkish police stations still have hand-cranked magnetos manufactured in a state-owned factory to administer shocks.[14]

Mains powered electric shock devices can be as simple as two bare wires pushed into an electrical outlet, with the other ends touched against the victim.[3,5] Some victims of torture describe more complex systems, such as their bare legs being tied to the metal legs of a chair through which they received shocks when the interrogating officer pressed a switch on his desk. Sometimes transformers are used to modify the AC wall current to one with lower potential. In some cases a fixed electrode was placed on one of the extremities, e.g. the big toe, and another electrode has been moved around to other parts of the body,[10] or a fixed electrode has been placed in each temporal region and a third one moved around.[3] The electrode can be attached to the target with a pincer, a clamp or a crocodile clip. In Latin America electric torture was applied while the person was immobilised on an iron bed ('La parilla').[10]

'I felt wires touching my neck and legs. Every time the wires touched my body, I shuddered. One time, the wires were placed on my genitals and he told me "You will not be able to have children."' 'In an other instance, I received electric shocks on my genitals while two interrogators stomped on my body. One stood on my chest and the other on my legs. The shock was so violent that the two interrogators fell to the ground.'[8]

The original battery driven electric shock batons delivering AC current were cattle prods used particularly in South America. They were modified in the 1970s for use in torture, the commonest being the 'Picana', which has an electrode shaped like a knitting needle.[3] Most often the point is used for the torture, but the pin can also be placed tangentially on the skin or connected to handcuffs. Many other types of electric shock baton have been developed since. One type is a 38 cm long baton with a battery driven generator operating as an induction coil to transform a current of low potential into a current of high potential. It has two round, slightly convex electrodes, 10 mm in diameter, placed in a distance of 7 mm at its top edge.[5,15]

In recent years, more and more sophisticated high-pulse and high-voltage stun weapons have been developed such as stun guns, stun shields, tasers, and remote controlled stun belts.[6,16] The current is transmitted directly to the body through two electrodes on the top edge of the stun gun, while the taser fires out wires which attach to clothing or skin with barbs and through which the electro-shock is carried to the target. The belt delivers a 50,000 V, 3–4 mA shock, which lasts 8 s and enter the body at the site of the electrodes near the kidneys. The electro-shock cannot be stopped once activated. The shield is placed over the victim and is made of a transparent type material with vertical and horizontal metal strips. It has two handles and between the handles a black box probably containing the battery. The Chinese manufacture an electric shock baton that was copied from one sent from the UK for sales purposes.

It has, however, often been difficult to obtain reliable information about the instruments used since the victims have been kept blindfolded during the torture. However, when the electric torture was applied, a sound was often heard. Sometimes victims of torture experience what feels to them like electric shocks from other forms of torture, such as water dripping on the head.

HISTORY

A detailed history of the electric torture is important since lesions can be absent or uncharacteristic, and a characteristic history may thus be the only support of the allegation of torture. Electric torture requires two body contacts (unless static electricity generators, e.g. as those manufactured for scalp massage are used). The locations of the body contacts and the shape of the electrodes are important information.

Electric torture can be applied to all parts of the body but has often been applied to sensitive parts, e.g. the genitals, the breasts, especially the nipples, the lips, gums, tongue, and teeth, and the throat, ears and eyes, including the cornea through the eyelids.[17] In order to increase the efficiency of the torture and to try to prevent detectable electric injuries, torturers often pour water or gels on the skin. Generally, the torturers appear to have specialised knowledge about how to use electricity on the human body in order to try to avoid objectively recognisable tissue damage and to keep the victim alive. Sometimes a medical doctor is present during the torture.

Electric current follows the shortest route between the two electrodes through tissue with the lowest resistance, i.e. blood vessels, muscles, and nerves. Among the symptoms is pain, often exquisitely pain, and since the muscles along the route of the electrical current are tetanically contracted, trembling, cramps or muscular paralysis may develop.[3,5] Victims have reported 'jumping' from the floor or chair when the electricity was applied.[8] A victim fastened to a bench by wrists and ankles felt as if his right leg and arm were being torn off when the electricity was switched on and he fainted.[10]

The muscular contraction may cause difficulties in breathing, dislocation of joints and fractures, the pain syncope. Henry Alleg[1] has reported his jaws being attached to the electrode by burning of the current, having a long wire forced into his mouth down into the throat. He could not open his mouth. If the current passes through the heart, cardiac arrest may follow.[18] While a choke baton with two closely placed electrodes primarily will influence the skin inducing pain and localised muscle contraction, the high-voltage stun weapons may, besides an exquisitely severe pain, cause immobilisation, self-defecation and self-urination since the current flow cannot be limited to the pathway between the electrodes.[6]

The use of electric torture more than most other types of torture suggests that torture is methodical. Thus a close correlation between stories concerning details in the use of electricity from victims with no prior contact with each other will heighten their value. The position of the victim and of the torturers during the torture, the clothing of the victim and a description of the room are among the useful information besides details about the instrument, the current and the number of electrodes as well as the number of shocks and their symptoms. Also information of what was said during the torture and whether there was a doctor present might be helpful.

SYMPTOMS FOLLOWING THE TORTURE

For some days after the torture the victim will have pain in the muscles from the tetanic contractions and the tears in the muscles, particularly if the shock was more than transient. Widespread muscular pain and tenderness, difficulty in standing and walking may persist for months. There is likely to be fear of future electric shocks, which may appear as hypervigilance and insomnia. In many cases this resolves once the victim is released, usually leaving persistent nightmares. In some cases this may develop into post-traumatic stress disorder.

Most of the sequelae of electrical torture are non-specific. They include damage to blood vessels, muscles, nerves, bone, and to the eyes and ears. If large amounts of energy are passing through the body, particularly via AC, thrombosis, oedema and tissue necrosis may develop. During the first 2 to 3 days after electric torture, the urine may contain myoglobin leaked from the blood because of damage to the muscles, and a red-brown discolouration of the urine may be observed.[11] Serum creatine kinase can be raised 2 to 3 weeks after electric torture. Differential diagnosis will be other types of muscle damage as blunt trauma. If a high concentration of myoglobin develops in the blood anuria may result.[19] Markedly reduced muscle strength may be found as well as lack of normal tendon reflexes. Permanent physical disability and loss of function may result. A total rupture of the right quadriceps muscle has been found $2\frac{1}{2}$ year after electric torture.[10] He walked with a limp. One victim reported violent swelling and wounds in his mouth.[3]

Cervical arthrosis has been observed 3 months after electric torture via an iron band clamped around the neck of a previously healthy 29-year-old man.[20] He complained of pain in the neck radiating to the hand, parasthesia of the fingers, stomach pain, and sleep disorders. He had painful and stiff neck muscles. Cervical arthrosis of C3–C4 and sequelae of a probably old fracture of the C3–C4 articular process was observed on X-ray.

A victim reported a pulsating tinnitus following electric torture to the auditory canals.[10] An inflamed eardrum was observed and later on a healed atrophic scar. Audiometry demonstrated a marked hearing loss.

Opacities were observed in the cornea 10 years after electric torture to the eyes influencing the vision.[17] Following a penetrating keratoplastic surgery, microscopic and electron microscopic changes of the removed tissue were observed, including dark deposits below the Bowman membrane.

ACUTE SKIN LESIONS

In some of the cases electric torture leaves acute lesions on the skin. The lesions may show an indication of electrically inflicted damage as described below. Since, however, a large part of the lesions heal up leaving no or insignificant scars, a characteristic history at a later examination of the acute lesions and their development until healing is important, a possible secondary infection included.

The lesions should be described by their localisation, symmetry, pattern, shape, size, colour and surface (e.g. scaly, bullous, crusty, necrotic, ulcerating) as well as by their periphery and demarcation in relation to the surrounding skin. The presence of other types of externally induced lesions and skin diseases should be described and possible differential diagnoses considered, self-infliction included.

Immediately following 'Picana' clusters and linear arrangements of 1–5 mm wide lesions covered by red-brown crusts, sometimes surrounded by a 1–2 mm broad erythematous zone with irregular and indistinct edges, may be seen.[10] Lesions in lines following a linear application of the electrodes may also be seen. Sometimes, according to the victims, electric torture left red lesions, occasionally with blisters, or pale lesions (necrosis?). [10] In addition, black spots and black pustules have been reported.[3] Well-demarcated, serpigineous lesions, measuring 1–2 cm across, with an irregular, narrow, elevated, peripheral zone and a central area containing several black spots, each measuring 1–2 mm, have also been observed (Figure 13.1).[18] A stun gun delivering 150,000 V has been reported to leave red marks which later on turned into black.[21] The lesions are usually located in non-symmetric areas of the skin.

An electric current causes, according to experimental studies on fully anaesthetised pigs using round, slightly convex electrodes measuring 12 mm in diameter and energy amounts from 6 to 285 J, specific electrical injuries, different from burn injuries, although some concomitant heat development occurs during the passage of the electric current.[22,23] Such heat development is particularly pronounced in cases with transfer of large amounts of energy as occurs during electrical accidents. While burn lesions following the transfer of energy via heated instruments are diffused, reflecting the shape of the instrument, their size, the amount of energy used, and often present a regular narrow zone of inflammation in the periphery, the lesions following electrical application may appear in segments within the influenced areas, the current selecting tissues with low resistance. The characteristic lesions following AC (50 and 8000 Hz) are 1–2 mm large brown crusty scales, while following DC a few mm large lesions or larger serpigineous lesions developed by confluence of smaller lesions may be seen. The lesions in the anode area are characterised by brown scales, in the

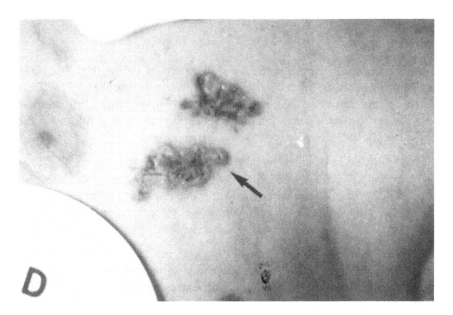

Figure 13.1 – Two well-demarcated serpigineous lesions measuring 1–2 cm across (arrow) from the chest wall of a 5-year-old girl shortly after electric injury. The lesions contain several circular black spots, each measuring about 1 mm in diameter. A similar lesion was present on the left arm[18]

cathode area by a central white necrosis and an irregular peripheral zone of inflamma-tion.[24,25] The brown scales represent deposition of iron from the electrode.

Usually, lesions following electric torture lack a regular narrow zone of inflammation in the periphery. The lesions contain too little necrotic tissue to induce a macroscop-ically visible inflammation. For lesions following 'Picana', insect bites might constitute a differential diagnose, but these are often accompanied by a red periphery because of dilated capillaries. Black, probably haemorrhagic lesions may indicate electrical influence since vessels are among the tissues with low resistance, and the presence of 1–2 mm large spots inside larger lesions together with a serpiginous periphery of the lesions are a further indication. Vasculitis or haemorrhagic herpes zoster might consti-tute a differential diagnosis. The location might be helpful since vasculitis chiefly is located to the lower extremities and symmetrical, sometimes more diffusely located, and herpes zoster to an area innervated by a single ganglion and unilateral.

SCARS

The scars are often non-specific, but a location, pattern, size or shape indicating external infliction may be able to support the history of electric torture to some degree. The presence of other types of scars, previous and present skin diseases, should be described and possible differential diagnoses considered. Clusters of round red macular cicatrices, about 1 mm in diameter, have been observed 4 weeks after 'Picana'.[26] Eight weeks later many of the scars had disappeared. The remaining scars were small, white or red-brown spots. The scars had no sequelae resulting from inflammatory reactions in their periphery as seen after burn, with heated instruments as a regular narrow hypertrophic or hyperpigmented zone (Figure 13.2).[27] Among the skin diseases leaving pigmented scars is lichen planus leaving about 2 mm large scars, but these are often quadratic. Electric torture has been reported to induce long-standing 6–8 mm large, irregular, red-brown, keloid scars on the helix of both ears.[28] Differential diagnosis might be a chondrodermatitis helicis, but this is usually covered by a scale, pale and painful. Linear cicatrices measuring 1×10 mm have been observed on the dorsum of fingers following electric torture with wires wrapped around the fingers 6 months previously, the shape and location indicating external infliction as reported.[5] Six months after the use of a 45 cm long stun gun with a screw 4 mm in diameter at its end and 12 small places where electricity also comes out from the lower part of its side, a sharply demarcated bluish line 1 mm across forming a complete circle 5 mm in diameter and a second mark of similar characteristics com-pleting only two-thirds of a circle were observed,[21] also indicating external infliction as described. Similar fractions of a narrow red ring have been seen in the days after defibrillation using 2736 V along the periphery of the pad.[29] In many cases, however, no signs of electric torture on the skin have been found. All suspected lesions should be photographed.

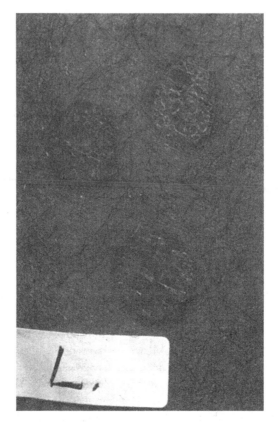

Figure 13.2 – Circular scars with an atrophic centre and a narrow, regular hyperpigmented zone in the periphery 1 year after alleged torture via an electrically heated, solid instrument the size and shape of a cigarette[27]. Reproduced with kind permission from Acta Dermato–Venerologica

HISTOLOGIC EXAMINATION OF SKIN LESIONS

If the victim agrees, a 3–4 mm punch biopsy in local anaesthesia might be helpful in supporting the allegation of electric torture.[30] Histologic examinations of skin biopsies are used as routine method in the diagnoses of skin diseases. Previously, only a few cases of electric torture have been studied histologically.[9,18,31] Only in one case, where lesions were excised 7 days after the injury, have alterations in the skin diagnostic of electrical injuries been observed (deposition of calcium salts on dermal fibres in viable tissue located around necrotic tissue) (Figure 13.3). In addition deposition of calcium salts on collagen fibres deep in dermis was observed (Figure 13.4). Lesions excised a few days after alleged electric torture showed segmental changes and deposits of calcium salts on cellular structures highly consistent with influence of an electric current, however not diagnostic since deposits of calcium salts on dermal fibres

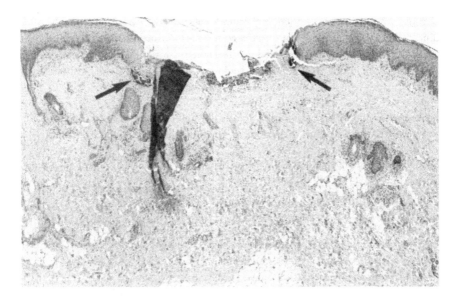

Figure 13.3 – Skin lesion from the chest wall of a 5-year-old girl 7 days after electric injury. An ulcer is seen that shows necrosis and inflammation in the upper part of dermis. Calcified collagen fibres appearing as small basophilic areas (arrows) are seen below the regenerated epidermis at the periphery of the lesion. Hematoxylin–eosin stain[18]

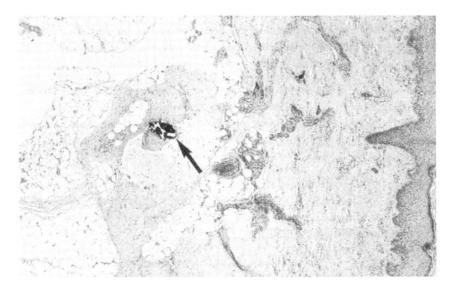

Figure 13.4 – Skin lesion of a 5-year-old girl 7 days after electric injury showing calcified collagen fibres appearing as a basophilic stained area (arrow) within the lower part of dermis. Hematoxylin–eosin stain[18]

were not observed. A biopsy taken 1 month after alleged electric torture showed a conical scar, 1–2 mm broad, with increased number of fibroblasts and tightly packed, thin collagen fibres, arranged parallel to the surface, consistent with but not diagnostic of electrical injury. No abnormal findings do not exclude the possible use of electric torture.

The biopsy should be placed in buffered formalin (Lillies's solution) and sections stained with hematoxylin–eosin and Alizarin red S (method appears from the Appendix).

The following alterations have been described after electrical injury of fully anaesthetised pigs.

Epidermal changes[23,32–34]

The changes are dependent on the kind of current applied and the amount of energy deposited. A large amount of energy will always produce ulceration and deep necrosis. Changes in epidermis suggestive of electrically induced damage are not likely to be found in a skin biopsy in such cases. Lower amounts of energy will on the other hand produce different changes in epidermis after AC and DC, and lesions after DC will have a different morphology in anode areas and cathode areas.

The lesions in cathode areas may be segmental or diffuse. Epidermis may contain vesicular nuclei, i.e. irregular and large nuclei with clear nucleoplasm, sometimes containing large, irregular clumps of chromatin. The cytoplasm may appear homogeneous with a pale or whitish staining reaction. Vesicular nuclei were also observed following injury via basic solutions in agreement with the basic pH present in the cathode area. Vesicular nuclei are only present a few days after the injury.

Anode lesions are often segmental. Metallic deposition in stratum corneum may be seen. The nuclei are usually small, with uniformly dispersed chromatin. The cytoplasm may appear homogeneous with an eosinophilic staining reaction. Similar alterations were observed following injury via acid solutions in agreement with the acid pH present in the anode area.

AC (50 and 8000 Hz) produces a morphology, that is a mixture of cathode and anode changes. In addition changes due to heat generation such as small defects lined by stretched, epidermal cells may be present in the epithelium. The cytoplasm may also be granular or fibrillar eosinophilic.

High-frequency AC (100,000 Hz) produces lesions almost exclusively due to heat generation. The characteristic changes are elongation of cells and nuclei ('streaming') and a fibrillar or granular eosinophilic cytoplasm, a morphology, which formerly and still in text books wrongly is considered characteristic of electrical injury. Exactly the same changes occur after a moderate heat injury to the skin.

Dermal changes[22,35-37]

The lesions following small amounts of energy appear as small cone-shaped necrotic segments following AC and larger necrotic segments following DC. Deposits of Alizarin red S positive calcium salts distinctly located to collagen and elastic fibres within viable tissue are seen 2 days after the injury in the cathode area in a narrow zone encircling the necrotic segment at some distance. In the following days, calcified foci are seen in increasing number and size as the collagen and elastic fibres situated superficially to those already containing calcium salts become calcified. At day 7 the calcified collagen fibres reach the regenerated epidermis. Three weeks after exposure, signs of transepidermal rejection of calcified material are seen, and 2 months after injury several small fractions of calcified collagen fibres are still present throughout a fibrotic dermis. Calcium deposits on collagen fibres following AC (50 Hz) are seen at day 7, but only by the use of larger, more concentrated amounts of energy than used for DC via pointed electrodes. Cellular alterations as those observed in epidermis can also be seen in sweat glands and vessel walls. Calcium deposits on cellular structures (sweat glands, hair follicles) are seen in heat lesions and more rarely in electrical lesions.

Diagnostic findings for electrical injury are

1. vesicular nuclei in epidermis, sweat glands and vessel walls (only one differential diagnosis: injuries via basic solutions);

2. deposits of calcium salts distinctly located to collagen and elastic fibres (the differential diagnosis, calcinosis cutis, is a rare disorder only found in 75 of 220,000 consecutive human skin biopsies, and the calcium deposits are usual massive without distinct location to collagen and elastic fibres).[18]

Typical findings for electrical injury are

1. lesions appearing in conical segments, often 1–2 mm large;

2. deposits of iron or copper on epidermis (from the electrode);

3. homogeneous cytoplasm in epidermis, sweat glands and vessel walls;

4. deposits of calcium salts on cellular structures in segmental lesions.

Where there are no abnormal histologic observations this does not exclude the possible use of electric torture.

HIGH-FREQUENCY ULTRASOUND OF SKIN LESIONS

This can be a useful non-invasive supplementary method since dermis and subcutaneous tissue are clearly distinguished in the ultrasound image,[38] and various pathological changes can be examined, e.g. the thickness of a scar and the presence of deposition of calcium salts, as it has been observed in the skin of patients with pseudo-xanthoma elasticum as extremely hyperechogenic areas (unpublished data). Thus this method could be useful to discover the location of calcium deposits in order to select an area for biopsy.

HISTOLOGIC EXAMINATION OF TISSUE FROM AREAS OTHER THAN THE SKIN

Sometimes it may be possible to observe changes in tissues removed from the path of the electric current, and examine it for histologic changes. The best example of this is of a child who had electrically induced cardiac arrest followed by cardiopulmonary resuscitation. The 5-year-old girl had been previously healthy and was declared dead a week later.[18] Deposits of calcium salts distinctly located to collagen fibres were observed within connective tissue adjacent to elastic arteries and peripheral nerves from the thoracic cavity.

APPENDIX

Preparing skin biopsies for the presence of calcium salts.

The biopsy is placed in buffered formalin: Lillies's solution.

Lillies's solution

Monosodium phosphate	4.52 g
Disodium phosphate ($2H_2O$)	8.10 g
Concentrated formalin solution (36% w/w)	108 g
Deionised water (to make a total of)	1000 ml

Alizarin red S staining

Reagents:

1. Alizarin red S – 0.5 g of Alizarin red S is dissolved in 45 ml of distilled water before adding with constant stirring 5 ml of a 100 times diluted solution of 28% NH_4OH solution. The pH must be in the range 6.3–6.5. If this is not the case adjustment may be made via adding more of the diluted NH_4OH solution or via adding distilled water. The staining solution must be thoroughly stirred prior to use. The solution will keep for at least 1 month.

2. Hydrochloric acid–ethanol solution – one drop of concentrated HCl plus 200 ml of 95% ethanol.

Procedure:

1. The histologic slides are deparaffinised and are treated with aqueous solutions with decreasing ethanol concentration until the slides appear clear. They are then treated shortly with running tap water and end up in distilled water. *Note:* No standing in water since calcium particles are slightly soluble in weakly acid solutions.
2. Staining with Alizarin red S solution for 2 min.
3. Rinsing with distilled water for 5 s.
4. Differentiation with hydrochloric acid–ethanol for 15 s.
5. Dehydration with several shifts of 99% ethanol followed by treatment with xylene until the slides appear clear. Then a cover slide is mounted.

Note: A control slide containing known calcium deposits is recommended.

Results:

1. Calcium particles appear orange-red.
2. Iron (not hemosiderin) is purple.

REFERENCES

1 Alleg H. The Question, 1958 (out of print)
2 Amnesty International: Report on Torture. London: Duckworth, 1975
3 Amnesty International: Danish Medical Group: Results of examination of 14 Argentinean torture victims. Frederiksborggade 1, DK-1360, Copenhagen K, Denmark, 1980, pp 1–56
4 Amnesty International: Report of an Amnesty International Mission to Spain 3–28 October 1979. London: Amnesty International Publications, 1980, pp 1–64
5 Amnesty International: Iraq. Evidence of Torture. London: Amnesty International Publications, 1981, pp 1–42
6 Amnesty International: USA. Cruelty in Control? – The stun belt and other electro-shock equipment in law enforcement. AI Index AMR 51/54/99, June 1999, pp 1–49
7 Berger P. Documentation of physical sequelae. Dan Med Bull 1980; 27: 215 216
8 Dillman JD, Bakri MA. Israel's use of electric shock torture in the interrogation of Palestinian detainees, Palestine Human Rights Information Center, Jerusalem 1991, pp 1–76
9 Öztop F, Lök V, Baykal T, Tunca M. Signs of electrical torture on the skin, in Human Rights Foundation of Turkey, Treatment and Rehabilitation Centers Report 1944, HRFT Publications 11: pp 97–104

10 Rasmussen OV. Medical aspects of torture (dissertation), University of Copenhagen, Danish Med Bull 1990; 37(suppl 1):1–88

11 Simpson MA. Methods of investigation allegations of electric shock torture: lessons from South Africa. Torture 1994; 4:27–29

12 Peters E. Torture. Philadelphia: University of Pennsylvania Press, 1996

13 Maran R. Torture: The Role of Ideology in the French–Algerian War. New York: Praeger, 1989

14 Forrest DM. Examination of the late physical after effects of torture. J Clin Forensic Med 1999; 6:4–13

15 Dyrhe-Poulsen P, Rasmussen L, Rasmussen OV. Investigation of an instrument of electrical torture (in Danish with an English summary). Ugeskr Læger 1977; 139:1054–1056

16 Wright S. The new trade in technologies of restraint and electroshock. In: Forrest D (ed.), A Glimpse of Hell: Reports of Torture Worldwide. London: Amnesty International/Cassell, 1996, pp 137–152

17 Perron-Buscail A, Lesueur L, Chollet P, Arne JL. Les brulures electriques corneennes: etude anatomo-clinique a propos d'un cas. J Fr Ophtalmol 1995; 18:384–386

18 Danielsen L, Karlsmark T, Thomsen HK, Thomsen JL, Balding LE. Diagnosis of electrical skin injuries. A review and a description of a case. Am J Forensic Med Pathol 1991; 12:222–226

19 Malik GH, Sirwal IA, Reshi AR et al. Acute renal failure following physical torture. Nephron 1993; 63:434–437

20 Smeulers J. Cervical arthrosis in a young man subjected to electric shock during imprisonment. Lancet 1975 (May 31):1249–1250

21 European Committee for the Prevention of Torture and Inhuman or Degrading Treatment or Punishment (CPT). Report to the Government of the Netherlands on the visit to the Netherlands Antilles carried out by the European Committee for the Prevention of Torture and Inhuman or Degrading Treatment or Punishment (CPT) from 7 to 11 December 1997 and Response of the Government of the Netherlands Antilles. CPT Inf. 1998; 17. [EN] (Part 1)

22 Karlsmark T, Thomsen HK, Danielsen L, Aalund O, Nielsen O, Nielsen KG, Genefke IK. Tracing the use of electrical torture. Am J Forensic Med Pathol 1984; 5:333–337

23 Thomsen HK. Electrically induced epidermal changes. A morphological study of porcine skin after transfer of low-moderate amounts of electrical energy (dissertation), University of Copenhagen. FADL, 1984, pp 1–78

24 Danielsen L, Thomsen HK, Nielsen O, Aalund O, Nielsen KG, Karlsmark T, Genefke IK. Electrical and thermal injuries in pig skin – evaluated and compared by light microscopy. Forensic Sci Int 1978; 12:211–225

25 Danielsen L. Skin changes following torture (in Danish with an English summary) Mdskr prakt lægeg April 1982, pp 193–209

26 Kjærsgaard AaR, Genefke IK. Torture in Uruguay and Argentina (in Danish with an English summary). Ugeskr Læger 1977; 139:1057–1059

27 Danielsen L, Berger P. Torture sequelae located to the skin. Acta Dermatovener (Stockholm) 1981; 61:43–46

28 Bork K, Nagel C. Long-standing pigmented keloid of the ears induced by electrical torture. J Am Acad Dermatol 1997; 36:490–491

29 Danielsen L, Gniadecka M, Thomsen HK, Pedersen F, Strange S, Nielsen KG, Petersen HD. Skin changes following defibrillation (unpublished data)

30 Aalund O, Danielsen L, Genefke I, Karlsmark T, Thomsen HK, Nielsen KG, Nielsen O. Diagnosis of electrical skin injuries. Video-tape, Copenhagen IRCT, Torture 1995; 5:34

31 Danielsen L, Karlsmark T, Thomsen HK. Diagnosis of skin lesions following electrical torture. Rom J Leg Med 1997; 15–20

32 Thomsen HK, Danielsen L, Nielsen O, Aalund O, Nielsen KG, Karlsmark T, Genefke IK. Early epidermal changes in heat- and electrically injured pig skin. A light microscopic study. Forensic Sci Int 1981; 17:133–143

33 Thomsen HK, Danielsen L, Nielsen O, Aalund O, Nielsen KG, Karlsmark T, Genefke IG, Christoffersen P. The effect of direct current, sodium hydroxide and hydrochloric acid on pig epidermis. A light microscopic and electron microscopic study. Acta Pathol Microbiol Immunol Scand Sect A 1983; 91:307–316

34 Jacobsen H. Electrically induced deposition of metal on the human skin. Forensic Sci Int 1997; 90:85–92

35 Karlsmark T, Danielsen L, Thomsen HK, Aalund O, Nielsen O, Nielsen KG, Johnson E, Genefke IK. Tracing the use of torture: electrically induced calcification of collagen in pig skin. Nature 1983; 301:75–78

36 Karlsmark T, Danielsen L, Aalund O, Thomsen HK, Nielsen O, Nielsen KG, Lyon H, Ammitsbøll T, Møller R, Genefke IK. Electrically-induced collagen calcification in pig skin. A histopathologic and histochemical study. Forensic Sci Int 1988; 39:163–174

37 Karlsmark T. Electrically induced dermal changes. A morphological study of porcine skin after transfer of low–moderate amounts of electrical energy (dissertation) University of Copenhagen. Dan Med Bull 1990; 37:507–520

38 Gniadecka M, Danielsen L. High-frequency ultrasound for torture-inflicted skin lesions. Acta Derm Venereol (Stockh) 1995; 75:375–376

14

RADIODIAGNOSTIC APPROACHES IN THE DOCUMENTATION OF TORTURE

R Semih Aytaçlar, Veli Lök

INTRODUCTION

Torture does not initially seem to appear within the scope of radiology. It is, therefore, necessary to have some specialized training and experience in applying diagnostic criteria.

Although the diagnostic results in general traumatology are considered to be quite successful, the lesions of torture must be interpreted in the light of events and their timing. Furthermore, lesions of torture tend to be specific to the area afflicted. It must always be stressed that the absence of lesions on investigation must never be considered to be evidence of absence of torture.

FORMS OF TORTURE AND RADIODIAGNOSTICS

Lesions of torture do not share the classical common features of general traumatology with which we are familiar. This is due to the way the lesions are caused. It is well known that systematic torture tends to be non-specific and torturers try to disguise the evidence.

Non-specific lesions can easily be overlooked if they are not related in the history of torture. Thus, it is important to note the site of lesion as well as the procedures leading to it. It is also important to ascertain the development of non-specific lesions with respect to time in relation to torture. In other words, knowing what to look for enhances the search and underlines the importance of three factors:[1,2]

1. the expected location of lesion,

2. the kind of specific procedure causing the lesion,

3. the time when the procedure took place.

These facts will not only avoid missing a non-specific finding but will also enable to relate the lesion to a specific procedure. Thus, it can be possible to identify acute, subacute and chronic lesions.

Radiological studies and scintigraphy can yield important information on signs and effects of torture. However, torture can be of one or more of the three main groups:

1. pharmacological,

2. psychological,

3. somatic.

The fundamental diagnostic role of radiology is in documenting recent somatic torture. However, although there is insufficient experience at present, it maybe possible to evaluate the haemodynamic effects of some types of pharmacological torture with Doppler ultrasound in future. Vascular effects of pharmacological agents are being evaluated with ultrasound (US) in numerous investigations which are beyond the scope of this study.[3–7] Therefore, US can well be utilized as to verify the effects of non-therapeutic pharmacological agents used in torture. This indicates the necessity for studies evaluating such effects.

Although it offers only limited applications, there are multiple studies suggesting the possibility of using functional magnetic resonance imaging (MRI) as supportive of US or images documenting long-term psychological effects of torture.[8–14] US studies present a similar potential.[15,16] Thus, transcranial US has revealed dynamic circulatory changes following visual and auditory stimulation reflecting past experiences among those exposed to long periods of stress. Present studies are investigating these changes in populations not exposed to similar conditions.[17,18] These studies could significantly contribute to documentation of psychological torture.

Systematic torture by political regimes varies according to geography as well as cultural, historical and customary relations. Torture regardless of its relation to the prevailing governments may well be unique with respect to civil or official organizations, as 'domuz bagi' (boar tie: after tying hands and feet together, a rope passing around the neck ties the hand to feet) reflects historical influences and local customs. Beatings are universal, although implements vary. Falaka, Palestinian suspension, electrical torture and anal assaults are among the most prevalent modes in Turkey. Specific criteria are available for diagnostic approaches to the various forms of somatic torture.

THE PRE-EXISTING LESION AND RADIODIAGNOSTICS

One of the fundamental problems is the existence of another pre-existing lesion leading to discovery of the lesion attributed to torture. A pre-existing lesion creates the following problems:

1. It can augment the visibility and the effects of specific forms of torture.

2. Its presence can cover-up the specific effects of torture.

3. Its effects can be mistaken for the effects of torture.

These problems are very important, since radiodiagnostics contribute to medico-legal evidence in cases of torture. As attribution of specific effects of tortures to an pre-existing lesion minimizes the medico-legal influence of non-specific findings to torture, and so can lead to mis-diagnosis and litigation.

PROFESSIONAL COLLABORATION AND SPECIFIC APPROACHES

Although the crude and primitive forms of torture provide a certain readiness for evaluation, the diagnostician must also be well equipped with information on other refined and systematic forms of torture. Therefore, the diagnostician needs to be not only knowledgeable and experienced but also in a productive collaboration with clinicians who are experienced in the field. A routine diagnostic approach may well make it impossible to recognize and evaluate an existing lesion. Thus, professionals engaged in radiodiagnosis of torture must have specific knowledge and experience. Otherwise, referral to more experienced radiodiagnostic centres is more practical. The professionals in these centres must be in close collaboration with the referring clinicians.

There is a need for further studies of the radiodiagnostic characteristics of specific lesions and their timing related to different forms of torture, and their medico-legal and forensic aspects. This process will require collaboration of international experts sharing their practice and knowledge, and also epidemiological analysis from rehabilitation centres with large numbers of patients. The reliability of such studies will increase due to technical generation of various diagnostic methods yielding a higher rate in the identification of lesions. Techniques such as MRI, computed tomography (CT) and US which significantly increase the reliability of radiodiagnosis have benefited from the present technological advances. Thus, detection of small lesions in soft tissues and bones has been substantially improved.

FORMS OF TORTURE AND CHOICE OF RADIODIAGNOSTIC TECHNIQUES

In clinical evaluation, documentation of the expected lesion depends on the proper choice of imaging. Radiodiagnostic techniques yield results varying in importance according to the type of expected lesion. Fundamental techniques used in radiodiagnosis are as follows:

1. direct examination with X-rays (conventional X-ray techniques),

2. computed tomography,

3. ultrasound,

4. magnetic resonance imaging,

5. scintigraphy.

X-rays

X-ray studies essentially involve direct X-ray films. In the evaluation of the peripheral small osseous structures, thickness of fine tissue and soft tissues, digital direct radiology, xeroradiographic approaches and even mammography can lead to important clues when in doubt. This group of studies are especially meaningful in ascertainment of lesions directed to the extremities and the trunk. They can be very useful when searching for fractures, fissures, deformity and foreign bodies in osseous structures.

The type of fracture can reveal important information on the force and its form of application. In this respect, soft tissue changes adjacent to the fracture or deformity as well as foreign bodies in the vicinity can also contribute information. The awareness of the forms of torture used can specify the cause of a lesion otherwise considered to be non-specific. Extension deformities can be followed up with these approaches during chronic stages.

Computed tomography

Both conventional and high resolution CT are very important in documenting a variety of lesions. CT is generally employed in lesions of soft tissues and the central nervous system. It can be very effective in revealing the timing and age of lesions by demonstrating small fissures and non-displaced fine fractures, and oedema and swelling of the adjacent soft tissues which cannot be recognized by direct X-rays. It can also show soft tissue changes, tissue atrophy, contractures and acute stage changes. High resolution CT can also help visualize fine haemorrhagic areas of lung parenchyma and rib fractures. It can also play an important role in determining the time of acute stages with accompanying soft tissue changes in acute lesions of the central nervous system.

Ultrasound

Contributions of US are generally considered in two areas:

1. morphologic,

2. functional.

Although US is primarily used for evaluation of muscles and joints, especially the shoulder joint, its contributions can be much wider depending on the skill of the applicator administering it. Insufficient documentation increases the possibility of mis-diagnosis as results may appear conclusive. However, results by less experienced operators can well serve as a document for more experienced specialist for the event later.

Contribution of conventional US varies according to its capacity for morphological evaluation. At present high channel probes with multifrequencies between 8 and 15 MHz can be more sensitive than CT and MRI in showing changes in cutaneous, subcutaneous, osseous and soft tissues as well as in muscles and joints. US sensitivity to pathology related to shoulder, knee and ankle joints, and related lesions of joints, tendons and adjacent soft tissues is usually higher than MRI. It is possible to demonstrate correctly muscle contusion and haematomas, subcutaneous contusion and haemorrhages, loss of uniformity of subcutaneous fat tissue, soft tissue micro- and macro-calcifications and foreign bodies with US. Traumatic changes and contusions of soft tissue in genitals, breast and perineum can be identified in detail with high resolution probes.

Furthermore, if the lesions are already located, cortical oedema, osteochondral injuries and small cortical discontinuities can be shown in superficial osseous lesions open to trauma much better than other approaches. Administration of US with these techniques can enable lesions of frequent beating such as falaka to be visualized. Sites of osseous lesions are usually proximal to the surface areas where torture was directed.

A second contribution is information on the perfusion of tissues identified by Doppler studies. Focal deficits of tissue perfusion and areas of reactive hyperaemia can be identified in injuries especially caused by cold (cold water and cold air). Findings of testicular torsion or of early detorsion can also be successfully demonstrated. It is also possible to demonstrate fracture, fissure, small osseous cortical discontinuities, neovascularization due to wound healing, or reactive periosteal callus formation in osteochondral injuries earlier and more precisely in comparison to direct X-rays or CT and MRI. However, in cases when there are no cortical injuries, verification of medullary and trabecular osseous changes is possible neither by classic nor by Doppler sonographic studies.

Perfusion problems of joint capsules in cases of inappropriate binding and forced extension can also be demonstrated with Doppler studies. Thus, alteration of triphasic flow to monophasic (secondary to hypoxia) in circumflex and geniculate arteries can indicate the locality and type of trauma. Oedema and traumatic reperfusion, and hyperaemia of sciatic and median nerves can be verified by both morphological studies with high resolution and Doppler studies. Findings of atrophy can also be verified in chronic stages.

Magnetic resonance imaging

Recently there have been significant advances in demonstration of acute and chronic lesions using MRI. Although it has similar applications with CT, it is more sensitive in many fields. MRI with Turbo STIR sequences, directed to the whole body can demonstrate general body trauma and identify lesions and areas needing detailed evaluation (see Figure 14.1). Unidentified lesions and those not causing any clinical complaints can also be visualized. Early stage cortical and medullary oedema and trabecular destructions can be much more readily demonstrated than CT. Minimal changes identified as bone bruise in pre-oedema stages can also be identified in osseous tissues. New special sequences which can verify these changes within hours are being developed and administered. Small millimetric cortical destructions, minimal oedematous changes of soft tissue, especially in series with fat suppression, and muscle contusion or strain injuries can also be identified.[19] The superiority of high resolution US depends on its success to demonstrate changes in all compartments of osseous tissue including tendon and ligaments covered by soft tissue and osseous structures. Lesions of the central nervous system, small areas of haemorrhage and traumatic perfusion

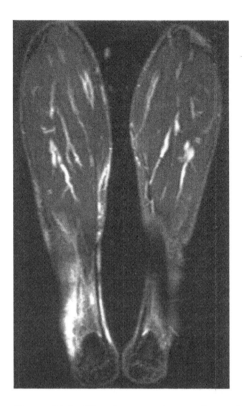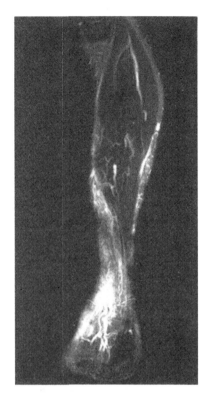

Figure 14.1 – Hyperintense oedema and contusion fields in the right ankle with Turbo STIR MRI after common beating

changes can generally be verified by FLAIR sequence, diffusion and perfusion studies in early stages. It is also possible to demonstrate chronic bone bruises and similar changes years after the trauma.

Scintigraphy

Scintigraphy is more sensitive in the demonstration of bone tissue lesions than classical radiological techniques. It allows observation of the effects years later. It is more cost effective than MRI, which can verify lesions in early stages. Fundamental events in revealing the pathology are osteoblastic activity and increased blood flow in tissues. In trauma not leading to fractures, bone metabolism and thus turnover is increased, and as trauma continues microfractures develop. The contribution of scintigraphy significantly increases in areas such as ribs, spinous processes and the scaphoid bone, which are hard to evaluate by direct X-rays. Thus, scintigraphy yields better results in trauma directed to thorax. Lesions such as epiphyseal separation or metaphyseal edge fractures which are easily missed can well be differentiated by the shape of epiphyseal plate and its visualization. Scintigraphy also provides advantages as a screening procedure following multiple traumata.

Another contribution of scintigraphy is that the activity of radioactive material changes in time. In acute stages positive results are obtained in 80% of the lesions within the first 24 h and 95% in 72 h. Chronic stage normally may last 1–2 years. However, in contrast to acute traumatic events results of torture may sometimes preserve the effects for as long as 10–15 years (see Figure 14.2). This indicates that the effects of the process causing the lesion may be well different in chronic stages.

Bone scintigraphy can show pathologic activity in the events that cause soft tissue destruction and local increase of vascularity even though there are no fractures of bone. Therefore, following torture, triphasic scintigraphy study of trauma site additional to total body scintigraphy will give information on increased vascularity of soft tissue (e.g., muscle tendon) with activity during the first two phases. Increased soft

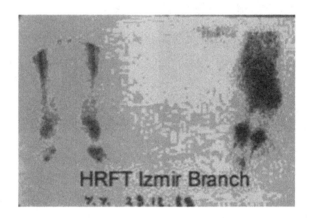

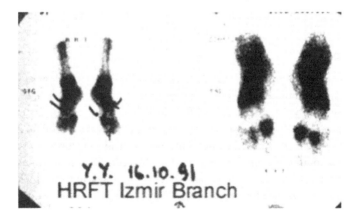

Figure 14.2 (a) and (b)

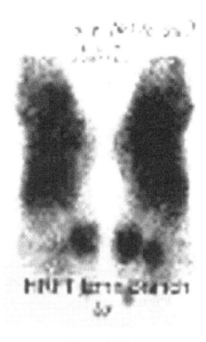

Figure 14.2(c)

Figure 14.2 – (a) Multiple areas of increased activity in structures of ankle and plantar bones during first scintigraphy 5 days later. (b) Persistence of osseous lesions in scintigraphy approximately 1 year later. (c) Apparent osseous activity even after 4 years. Such findings usually disappear within 1–2 years after acute trauma in contrast to their persistence for many years after torture

tissue vascularity following torsion of external genitalia and electrical shocks can often lead to clear evidence of torture.

Probability of positivity increases within time following trauma since it induces osteoblastic activity. Therefore, in this respect a negative scintigraphy during the first 48–72 h being positive 1 week later can well be a clue and indicate to torture. This positivity can continue up to 15 years in especially falaka due to its procedural characteristics. Specificity of scintigraphic findings following single impacts and multiple impacts on the same area differentiates them and verifies type of torture. Repetitive impact on the same area in bone regions close to body surface gives similar results.[20–23] Thus, in cases of common beating scintigraphy can give positive results.

Finally, in the event that direct X-rays are insufficient, scintigraphy must be administered. However, one must keep in mind that similar results can be obtained in people who are frequently exposed to repetitive trauma as in the case of accidents in sports, ankle sprains and commando training. Localization of findings and typical characteristics of activity areas can help in differentiation.

APPROACHES ACCORDING TO FORM OF TORTURE[1,21–30]

Common beating

- Blows to face and jaws result in soft tissue lesions, haematomas (especially those to sinuses) and fractures. Temporomandibular joint subluxation or joint disc injuries can well be verified by MRI.

- Clavicle, elbow, forearm and crural fractures or injuries can be demonstrated by scintigraphy or MRI in early stages.

Falaka

- Fractures are frequent following severe falaka. In early stages as oedema withdraws, pes planus can appear as connective tissues, fascia and tendons elongate. Closed compartment syndrome may develop. Haematomas, oedema and facial rupture injuries can be shown.

- MRI and high resolution US can yield important information on soft tissue changes and their evolution.

Electrical torture

- Cervical spasm and disruption of lordosis is common. Clavicle, rib and spinal process fractures are seen and although rarely osteonecrosis can develop.

- Scintigraphy can be used for general screening. CT can be useful in suspicious areas. MRI may significantly contribute to early diagnosis of osteonecrosis.

- Jaw fractures and teeth dislocations are common following electric shocks to the mouth and tongue.

Nail torture

- X-rays can sometimes verify when metallic tools are used for probing the nail bed.
- Findings related to soft tissue changes, haematoma, oedema and fractures can be demonstrated.

Puncture wounds

- US can verify closed haematoma and perforations in the acute stage.
- X-rays can often show metallic traces in soft tissue.

Suspension

Injuries of connective tissues, ligaments, tendons, axillary and brachial plexuses, axillary oedema and haematomas can be demonstrated by high resolution US and MRI directed to plexuses.

Others

- Depending on the geographic regions, squeezing and crushing directed to fingers (finger torture) and carpal regions may show fractures and amputations of finger or hand.

- Peripheral perfusion deficiencies resulting from pressure are verified by Doppler US.

- Aspiration pneumonias resulting from submersion are frequent and can be recognized by direct X-rays.

- Organ lacerations and haemorrhage can be verified by US, MRI and CT.

- Radio-opaque material placed in rectum are shown with X-rays. MRI can verify non-opaque and especially organic materials.

- Ulceration and haemorrhage of the stomach due to stress can be observed in chronic stages.

- Joint and other connective tissue deformities are shown with X-rays or MRI.

- Peripheral nerve ossification and pathology as myositis ossificans of muscles and soft tissues are shown with US and X-rays.

EVALUATION OF FINDINGS

- Evaluations of findings obtained from imaging techniques must consider forms of torture and their frequency as to their geographic, ethnic and cultural origins.

- Plantar oedema, plantar fascia injuries, metacarpal and phalanx fractures indicate falaka. Foreign bodies in nail bed, abdominal and thoracic subcutaneous tissue indicate specific types of torture. Brachial and axillary plexus injuries, axillary oedema and haematoma, connective tissue and bone injuries directed to this region are findings of falaka.

- Distortion of cervical axis, fractures of vertebral processes, jaw fractures involving teeth, soft tissue changes and accompanying rib fractures indicate to torture with electrical current (E-torture).

- In scintigraphy, activity of bone for more than 2 years may differentiate acute trauma from that due to torture.

CONCLUSION

Radiodiagnostic techniques provide a wide array of effective instruments in documentation and verification of torture, although the absence of findings on investigation is never significant. The fundamental problem here is contribution of the evaluation of findings from this different perspective to questions put forth by forensic medicine. Verification of lesions establishment of their relation with forms of torture and their timing certainly necessitates related knowledge, experience and further studies. In this respect, accumulation of knowledge and its specificity to somatic torture is expanding to other modes as well with present technology.

REFERENCES

1 Vogel H. Gewalt im Röntgenbild (X-ray diagnosis of violence). Landsberg: Befunde zu Krieg, Folter und Verbrechen ecomed, 1997
2 Diagnostic Imaging Europe: Imaging helps unveil torture's dark secrets. Diag Imaging Eur November 1999
3 Manno EM, Gress DR, Ogilvy CS, Stone CM, Zervas NT. The safety and efficacy of cyclosporine A in the prevention of vasospasm in patients with Fisher grade 3 subarachnoid hemorrhages: a pilot study. Neurosurgery 1997; 40(2): 289–293
4 Lennard N, Smith JL, Hayes P, Evans DH, Abbott RJ, London NJ, Bell PR, Naylor AR. Transcranial Doppler directed dextran therapy in the prevention of carotid thrombosis: three hour monitoring is as effective as six hours. Eur J Vasc Endovasc Surg 1999; 17(4):301–305
5 Sullivan JT, Becker PM, Preston KL, Wise RA, Wigely FM, Testa MP, Jasinski DR. Cocaine effects on digital blood flow and diffusing capacity for carbon monoxide among chronic cocaine users. Am J Med 1997; 102(3):232–238
6 Kanamaru K, Waga S, Kuga Y, Nakamura F, Kamata N. Transcranial Doppler pattern after intracarotid papaverine and prostaglandin E1 incorporated in lipid microsphere in patients with vasospasm. Neurol Med Chir (Tokyo) 1998; 38(suppl):152–155
7 Corbett SA, McCarthy ID, Batten J, Hukkanen M, Polak JM, Hughes SP. Nitric oxide mediated vasoreactivity during fracture repair. Clin Orthop 1999; 365:247–253
8 Mazurchuk R, Glaves D, Raghavan D. Magnetic resonance imaging of response to chemotherapy in orthotopic xenografts of human bladder cancer. Clin Cancer Res 1997; 3(9):1635–1641
9 Martì Bonmatì L, Dosd R, Ronchera Oms CL, Casillas C. Dose effect of dicyclomine on the reduction of peristaltic artifacts on MRI of the abdomen. Abdom Imaging 1999; 24(4):336–339
10 Yetkin FZ, Swanson S, Fischer M, Akansel G, Morris G, Mueller W, Haughton V. Functional MR of frontal lobe activation: comparison with Wada language results. Am J Neuroradiol 1998; 19(6):1095–1098
11 Hedera P, Wu D, Collins S, Lewin JS, Miller D, Lerner AJ, Klein S, Friedland RP. Sex and electroencephalographic synchronization after photic stimulation

predict signal changes in the visual cortex on functional MR images. Am J Neuroradiol 1998; 19(5):853–857

12 Yousem DM, Maldjian JA, Hummel T, Alsop DC, Geckle RJ, Kraut MA, Doty RL. The effect of age on odor-stimulated functional MR imaging. Am J Neuroradiol 1999; 20(4):600–608

13 Yurgelun Todd DA, Renshaw PF. Applications of functional MR imaging to research in psychiatry. Neuroimaging Clin N Am 1999; 9(2):295–308

14 Braus DF, Ende G, Weber Fahr W, Sartorius A, Krier A, Hubrich Ungureanu P, Ruf M, Stuck S, Henn FA. Antipsychotic drug effects on motor activation measured by functional magnetic resonance imaging in schizophrenic patients. Schizophrenia Res 1999; 39(1):19–29

15 Droupy S, Hessel A, BenoÖt G, Blanchet P, Jardin A, Giuliano F. Assessment of the functional role of accessory pudendal arteries in erection by transrectal color Doppler ultrasound. J Urol 1999; 162(6):1987–1991

16 Schmidt P, Krings T, Willmes K, Roessler F, Reul J, Thron A. Determination of cognitive hemispheric lateralization by 'functional' transcranial Doppler cross-validated by functional MRI. Stroke 1999; 30(5):939–945

17 Stoll M, Hamann GF, Mangold R, Huf O, Winterhoff Spurk P. Emotionally evoked changes in cerebral hemodynamics measured by transcranial Doppler sonography. J Neurol 1999; 246(2):127–133

18 Kadojic D, Demarin V, Kadojic M, Mihaljevic I, Barac B. Influence of prolonged stress on cerebral hemodynamics. Coll Antropol 1999; 23(2): 665–672

19 Hayes E. MRI illustrates history of torture. Diag Imaging Eur 1997; 13(4):17

20 Lök V, Tunca M, Kumanlioglu K, Kapkin E, Dirik G. Bone scintigraphy as clue to previous torture. Lancet 1991; 337:846–847

21 Lök V, Tunca M, Kapkin E et al. Bone scintigraphy as an evidence of previous torture: evidenced of 62 patients. Human Rights Foundation of Turkey (HRFT) treatment and rehabilitation centres report, 1994. Ankara: HRFT publications 1995, pp 91–96

22 Mirzaei S, Knoll P, Lipp RW, Wenzel T, Koriska K, Köhn H. Bone scintigraphy in screening of torture survivors. Lancet 1998; 352(9132):949–951

23 Tunca M, Lök V. Bone scintigraphy in screening of torture survivors. Lancet 1998; 352(9143):1859

24 Akcam T, Die 'Normalitat' der folter (Zur analyse eines herrschaftsmittels) Hrsg.: reemtsma, Junius Verlag GmbH Hamburg 1991, pp 155–186

25 Amnesty International: Report on Torture, revised edn. London: Amnesty International Publications, 1975

26 Amnesty International: Evidence of torture: Studies by the Amnesty International Danish Medical Group. London: Amnesty International Publication, 1977

27 Rasmussen OV, Lunde I. Evaluation of investigation of 200 torture victims. Dan Med Bull 1980; 27:241–243

28 Rasmussen OV. Medical Aspects of Torture. Kopenhagen: Laegeforemingens Forlag 1990, pp 1–85

29 Rasmussen OV, Marcussen H. Somatic consequences of torture. Manedskr Prakt Laegegern 1982; 111:124–140

30 Lucas CE. Stress ulceration: the clinical problem. World J Surg 1991; 5:139–151

INDEX

interviews using interpreters 92–95
objectives 78–79
risks of 79–90

W

whistleblowing, by health professionals 66–67
World Medical Association Declaration of
Tokyo

definition of torture 2
medical ethics and torture 8–9
World Psychiatric Association, statement on
ethics and torture 9

X

X-ray imaging, for evaluation of torture
210–211